PLANS OF CARE FOR SPECIALTY PRACTICE

Gerontological Nursing

JOAN F. NEEDHAM, MS, RNC
Director of Education
DeKalb County Nursing Home
DeKalb, Illinois

series editor
KATHY V. GETTRUST, RN, BSN
Case Manager
Midwest Medical Home Care
Milwaukee, Wisconsin

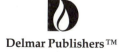

Delmar Publishers™

I(T)P™ An International Thomson Publishing Company

Albany • Bonn • Boston • Cincinnati • Detroit • London • Madrid • Melbourne
Mexico City • New York • Pacific Grove • Paris • San Francisco • Singapore • Tokyo
Toronto • Washington

NOTICE TO THE READER

Publisher does not warrant or guarantee any of the products described herein or perform any independent analysis in connection with any of the product information contained herein. Publisher does not assume, and expressly disclaims, any obligation to obtain and include information other than that provided to it by the manufacturer.

The reader is expressly warned to consider and adopt all safety precautions that might be indicated by the activities herein and to avoid all potential hazards. By following the instructions contained herein, the reader willingly assumes all risks in connection with such instructions.

The publisher makes no representations or warranties of any kind, including but not limited to, the warranties of fitness for particular purpose or merchantability, nor are any such representations implied with respect to the material set forth herein, and the publisher takes no responsibility with respect to such material. The publisher shall not be liable for any special, consequential, or exemplary damages resulting, in whole or in part, from the readers' use of, or reliance upon, this material.

Cover Illustration: Jeanne A. Benas

Delmar Staff

Publisher: David C. Gordon
Acquisitions Editor: Patricia E. Casey
Developmental Editor: Elena M. Mauceri
Senior Project Editor: Mary P. Robinson

Production Coordinator: Barbara A. Bullock
Art and Design Coordinator: Mary E. Siener
Editorial Assistant: Tonjia Herman

COPYRIGHT © 1995 by Delmar Publishers
a division of International Thomson Publishing Inc.

The ITP logo is a trademark under license.

Printed in the United States of America

For more information, contact:

Delmar Publishers
3 Columbia Circle, Box 15015
Albany, NY 12212-5015

International Thomson Publishing Europe
Berkshire House 168-173
High Holborn
London, WC1V 7AA
England

Thomas Nelson Australia
102 Dodds Street
South Melbourne, 3205
Victoria, Australia

Nelson Canada
1120 Birchmont Road
Scarborough, Ontario
Canada, M1K 5G4

International Thomson Editores
Campos Eliseos 385, Piso 7
Col Polanco
11560 Mexico D F Mexico

International Thomson Publishing GmbH
Konigswinterer Strasse 418
53227 Bonn
Germany

International Thomson Publishing Asia
221 Henderson Road
#05-10 Henderson Building
Singapore 0315

International Thomson Publishing Japan
Hirakawacho Kyowa Building, 3F
2-2-1 Hirakawacho
Chiyoda-ku, Tokyo 102
Japan

RC954
.N339
1995

1 2 3 4 5 6 7 8 9 10 XXX 00 99 98 97 96 95 94

Library of Congress Cataloging-in-Publication Data

Needham, Joan Fritsch.
  Gerontological nursing / Joan F. Needham
    p. cm. — (Plans of care for specialty practice)
  Includes index.
  ISBN 0-8273-6226-9
  1. Geriatric nursing. 2. Nursing care plans. I. Title. II. Series.
  [DNLM: 1. Geriatric Nursing. WY 152 N374ga 1994]
RC954.N339 1994
610.73 65—dc20
DNLM/DLC for Library of Congress   94-25559
                                                                        CIP

DEDICATION

This book is dedicated to the memory of my mother, Helen Fritsch.

TABLE OF CONTENTS

PREFACE

There are almost 32 million persons over 65 years of age in this country. It is anticipated that this number will double in the next 40 years. Data from the U.S. Department of Health and Human Services indicate that most older persons have at least one chronic condition and many have multiple conditions. Older people account for 45% of all days of care in hospitals.

These figures represent a tremendous need for nurses who are knowledgeable in caring for the elderly. Gerontological nursing is practiced in hospitals, long-term care facilities, personal homes, clinics, and adult day care centers. Elderly patients are unique. They are experiencing age-related physiological and functional changes. When these changes are compounded with a chronic, disabling illness, the risk factors for complications increase: infection, injury, trauma, aspiration, disuse syndrome, impaired skin integrity, and impaired physical mobility, to name a few.

Psychosocial alterations abound in persons in this age group. They have frequently undergone many losses and need nursing encouragement and support. However, these individuals are also survivors. In planning care, it is important to identify their strengths as well as their problems. The challenge to the nurse is great. Interventions require creativity, patience, and caring.

The theoretical framework for gerontological nursing is based on the premise that quality of life is dependent on the patient's need fulfillment, problem resolution, and self-determination. The essence of gerontological nursing is not necessarily to increase the length of life but to assist each person in fulfilling an optimal potential throughout life.

This book is written for the nurse who is responsible for provision of care to elderly persons. An attempt has been made to generate interventions that are appropriate for any setting where care is rendered. Emphasis has been given to problems associated with chronic illnesses frequently seen among the elderly population. Few diseases are unique to this age group, but as people live longer, they are statistically at greater risk for acquiring these diseases.

The interdisciplinary approach is a vital foundation for gerontological nursing. The patient's problems are complex and can be fully resolved only by utilizing team strategies. Care planning is most successful when completed at the interdisciplinary care planning conference.

Abbreviations used in this book can be found on the inside front cover, and the standards of gerontological nursing follow the series introduction. There are four appendices at the end of the book. Appendix A contains information relative to aging changes. Refer to this appendix often for a frame of reference for planning care. Elderly people are at risk for injury and trauma, and Appendix B provides an environmental assessment to reduce these risks. Appendix C includes suggestions for teaching elderly patients. The mini mental status examination is referred to frequently and is found in Appendix D. Clinical clips and tables are scattered throughout the chapters for additional information.

It is the hope of this author that nurses in all settings will find this book to be helpful in planning the care of their patients.

ACKNOWLEDGMENTS

As this book comes to a close, many individuals come to mind who continue to support me as I proceed with my writing projects for Delmar Publishers. I wish to thank Beth Williams, Health Sciences Editor, and Kathy Gettrust, Series Editor, for giving me the opportunity to participate in this series. I thank Elena Mauceri, Developmental Editor, and Administrative Editor, Patricia Casey, for their patience and assistance in preparing the manuscript. My husband, my daughters and their families, our extended family, and my friends and coworkers are sincerely appreciated for their ongoing interest, encouragement, and consideration.

SERIES INTRODUCTION

Scientific and technological developments over the past several decades have revolutionized health care and care of the sick. These rapid and extensive advancements of knowledge have occurred in all fields, necessitating an ever-increasing specialization of practice. For nurses to be effective and meet the challenge in today's specialty settings, the body of clinical knowledge and skill needs to continually expand. *Plans of Care for Specialty Practice* has been written to aid the practicing nurse in meeting this challenge. The purpose of this series is to provide comprehensive, state-of-the-art plans of care and associated resource information for patient situations most commonly seen within a specialty that will serve as a standard from which care can be individualized. These plans of care are based on the profession's scientific approach to problem solving—the nursing process. Though the books are written primarily as a guide for frontline staff nurses and clinical nurse specialists practicing in specialty settings, they have application for nursing students as well.

DOCUMENTATION OF CARE

The Joint Commission on Accreditation of Healthcare Organizations (JCAHO) assumes authority for evaluating the quality and effectiveness of the practice of nursing. In 1991, the JCAHO developed its first new nursing care standards in more than a decade. One of the changes brought about by these new standards was the elimination of need for every patient to have a handwritten or computer-generated care plan in his or her chart detailing all or most of the care to be provided. The Joint Commission's standard that describes the documentation requirements stipulates that nursing assessments, identification of nursing diagnoses and/or patient care needs, interventions, outcomes of care, and discharge planning be permanently integrated into the clinical record. In other words, the nursing process needs to be documented. A separate care plan is no longer needed; however, planning and implementing care must continue as always, but using whatever form of documentation that has been approved by an institution. *Plans of Care for Specialty Practice* can be easily used with a wide variety of approaches to documentation of care.

ELEMENTS OF THE PLANS OF CARE

The chapter title is the presenting situation, which represents the most commonly seen conditions/disorders treated within the specialty setting. It may be a medical diagnosis (e.g., diabetes mellitus), a syndrome (e.g., acquired immunodeficiency syndrome), a surgical procedure (e.g., mastectomy), or a diagnostic/therapeutic procedure (e.g., thrombolytic therapy).

An opening paragraph provides a definition or concise overview of the presenting situation. It describes the condition and may contain pertinent physiological/psychological bases for the disorder. It is brief and not intended to replace further investigation for comprehensive understanding of the condition.

Etiologies

A listing of causative factors responsible for or contributing to the presenting situation is provided. This may include predisposing diseases, injuries or trauma, surgeries, microorganisms, genetic factors, environmental hazards, drugs, or psychosocial disorders. In presenting situations where no clear causal relationship can be established, current theories regarding the etiology may be included.

Clinical Manifestations

Objective and subjective signs and symptoms that describe the particular presenting situation are included. This information is revealed as a result of a health history and physical assessment and becomes part of the data base.

Clinical/Diagnostic Findings

This component contains possible diagnostic tests and procedures that might be done to determine abnormalities associated with a particular presenting situation. The name of the diagnostic procedure and the usual abnormal findings are listed.

Nursing Diagnosis

The nursing management of the health problem commences with the planning care phase of the nursing process. This includes obtaining a comprehensive history and physical assessment, identification of the nursing diagnoses, expected outcomes, interventions, and discharge planning needs.

Diagnostic labels identified by NANDA through the Tenth National Conference in April 1992 are being used throughout this series (based on North American Nursing Diagnosis Association (1992). *NANDA Nursing Diagnoses: Definitions and Classification 1992–1993*. Philadelphia: NANDA.). We have also identified new diagnoses not yet on the official NANDA list. We endorse NANDA's recommendation for nurses to develop new nursing diagnoses as the need arises and we encourage nurses using this series to do the same.

"Related to" Statements

"Related to" statements suggest a link or connection to the nursing diagnosis and provide direction for identifying appropriate nursing interventions. They have sometimes been termed contributing factors, causes, or etiologies. There is frequently more than one "related to" statement for a given diagnosis. For example, change in job, marital difficulties, and impending surgery may all be "related to" the patient's nursing diagnosis of "Anxiety."

There is disagreement at present regarding inclusion of pathophysiologic/medical diagnoses in the list of "related to" statements. Frequently, a medical diagnosis does not provide adequate direction for nursing care. For example, the nursing diagnosis of "Chronic Pain" related to rheumatoid arthritis does not readily suggest specific nursing interventions. It is more useful for the nurse to identify specific causes of the chronic pain, such as inflammation, swelling, and fatigue; these in turn suggest more specific interventions. In cases where the medical diagnosis provides the best available information, as occurs with the more medically oriented diagnoses such as "Decreased Cardiac Output" or "Impaired Gas Exchange," the medical terminology is included.

Defining Characteristics

Data collection is frequently the source for identifying defining characteristics, sometimes called signs and symptoms or patient behaviors. These data, both subjective and objective, are organized into meaningful patterns and used to verify the nursing diagnosis. The most commonly seen defining characteristics for a given diagnosis are included and should not be viewed as an all-inclusive listing.

Risk Factors

Nursing diagnoses designated as high risk are supported by risk factors that direct nursing actions to reduce or prevent the problem from developing. Since these nursing diagnoses have not yet occurred, risk factors replace the listing of actual defining characteristics and "related to" statements.

Patient Outcomes

Patient outcomes are observable behaviors or data that measure changes in the condition of the patient after nursing treatment. They are objective indicators of progress toward prevention of the development of high-risk nursing diagnoses or resolution/modification of actual diagnoses. Like other elements of the plan of care, patient outcome statements are dynamic and must be reviewed and modified periodically as the patient progresses. Assigning realistic "target or evaluation dates" for evaluation of progress toward outcome achievement is crucial. Since there are so many considerations involved in when the outcome could be achieved (e.g., varying lengths of stay, individual patient condition), these plans of care do not include evaluation dates; the date needs to be individualized and assigned using the professional judgment and discretion of the nurse caring for the patient.

Nursing Interventions

Nursing interventions are the treatment options/actions the nurse employs to prevent, modify, or resolve the nursing diagnosis. They are driven by the "related to" statements and risk factors and are selected based on the outcomes to be achieved. Treatment options should be chosen only if they apply realistically to a specific patient condition. The nurse also needs to determine frequencies for each intervention based on professional judgment and individual patient need.

We have included independent, interdependent, and dependent nursing interventions as they reflect current practice. We have not made a distinction between these kinds of interventions because of institutional differences and increasing independence in nursing practice. The interventions that are interdependent or dependent will require collaboration with other professionals. The nurse will need to determine when this is necessary and take appropriate action. The interventions include assessment, therapeutic, and teaching actions.

Rationale

The rationale provides a scientific explanation or theoretical base for the intervention; interventions can then be selected more intelligently and actions can be tailored to each individual's needs.

The rationales provided may be used as a quick reference for the nurse unfamiliar with the reason for a given intervention and as a tool for patient education. These rationales may include principles, theory, and/or research findings from current literature. The rationales are intended as reference information and, as such, should not be transcribed into the permanent patient record. A rationale is not provided when the intervention is self-explanatory.

Discharge Planning/Continuity of Care

Because stays in acute care hospitals are becoming shorter due to cost-containment efforts, patients are frequently discharged still needing care; discharge planning is the process of anticipating and planning for needs after discharge. Effective discharge planning begins with admission and continues with ongoing assessment of the patient and family needs. Included in the discharge planning/continuity of care section are suggestions for follow-up measures, such as skilled nursing care; physical, occupational, speech, or psychiatric therapy; spiritual counseling; social service assistance; follow-up appointments; and equipment/supplies.

References

A listing of references appears at the conclusion of each plan of care or related group of plans. The purpose of the references is to cite specific work used and to specify background information or suggestions for further reading. Citings provided represent the most current nursing theory and/or research bases for inclusion in the plans of care.

Clinical Clips

Interspersed throughout the books are brief pieces of information related to the particular specialty. The intent is to blend some concept or theory tidbits with the practical nature of the books. This information not only may enrich the nurse's knowledge base but also may be used in the dissemination of patient education information.

A WORD ABOUT FAMILY

The authors and editors of this series recognize the vital role that family and/or other significant people play in the recovery of a patient. Isolation from the family unit during hospitalization may disrupt self-concept and feelings of security. Family members, or persons involved in the patient's care, must be included in the teaching to ensure that it is appropriate and will be followed. In an effort to constrain the book's size, the patient outcome, nursing intervention, and discharge planning sections usually do not include reference to the family or other significant people; however, the reader can assume that they are to be included along with the patient whenever appropriate.

ACKNOWLEDGMENTS

Any undertaking of the magnitude of this series becomes the concern of many people. I would specifically like to thank all of the very capable nursing specialists who authored or edited the individual books. Their attention to providing state-of-the-art information in a quick, usable form will provide the reader with current reference information for providing excellent patient care.

Special thanks also goes to my friend, Mark Gregory, for his clever coinage of the term "clinical clips."

The editorial staff, particularly Patricia E. Casey and Elisabeth F. Williams, and production people at Delmar Publishers have been outstanding. Their frank criticism, comments, and encouragement have improved the quality of the series.

Finally, but most importantly, I wish to thank my husband, John, and children, Katrina and Allison, for their sacrifices and patience during yet another publishing project.

Kathy V. Gettrust
Series Editor

STANDARDS OF GERONTOLOGICAL NURSING PRACTICE

The standards as defined by the American Nurses' Association call for quality care at a level beyond that required by minimal regulatory standards. The standards apply to gerontological nurses in all functional areas across all settings. The standards are included here so that gerontological nurses will use them as a model for professional practice.

STANDARD I. ORGANIZATION OF GERONTOLOGICAL NURSING SERVICES

All gerontological nursing services are planned, organized, and directed by a nurse executive. The nurse executive has baccalaureate or master's preparation and has experience in gerontological nursing and administration of long-term care services or acute-care services for older clients.

STANDARD II. THEORY

The nurse participates in the generation and testing of theory as a basis for clinical decisions. The nurse uses theoretical concepts to guide the effective practice of gerontological nursing.

STANDARD III. DATA COLLECTION

The health status of the older person is regularly assessed in a comprehensive, accurate, and systematic manner. The information obtained during the health assessment is accessible to and shared with appropriate members of the interdisciplinary health care team, including the older person and family.

STANDARD IV. NURSING DIAGNOSIS

The nurse uses health assessment data to determine nursing diagnoses.

STANDARD V. PLANNING AND CONTINUITY OF CARE

The nurse develops the plan of care in conjunction with the older person and appropriate others. Mutual goals, priorities, nursing approaches, and measures in the care plan address the therapeutic, preventive, restorative, and rehabilitative needs of the older person. The care plan helps the older person attain and maintain the highest level of health, well-being, and quality of life achievable as well as a peaceful death. The plan of care facilitates continuity of care over time as the client moves to various care settings and is revised as necessary.

STANDARD VI.   INTERVENTION

The nurse, guided by the plan of care, intervenes to provide care to restore the older person's functional capabilities and to prevent complications and excess disability. Nursing interventions are derived from nursing diagnoses and are based on gerontological nursing theory.

STANDARD VII.   EVALUATION

The nurse continually evaluates the client's and family's responses to interventions in order to determine progress toward goal attainment and to revise the data base, nursing diagnoses, and plan of care.

STANDARD VIII. INTERDISCIPLINARY COLLABORATION

The nurse collaborates with other members of the health care team in the various settings in which care is given to the older person. The team meets regularly to evaluate the effectiveness of the care plan for the client and family and to adjust the plan of care to accommodate changing needs.

STANDARD IX.   RESEARCH

The nurse participates in research designed to generate an organized body of gerontological nursing knowledge, disseminates research findings, and uses them in practice.

STANDARD X.   ETHICS

The nurse uses the code for nurses established by the American Nurses' Association as a guide for ethical decision making in practice.

STANDARD XI.   PROFESSIONAL DEVELOPMENT

The nurse assumes responsibility for professional development and contributes to the professional growth of interdisciplinary team members. The nurse participates in peer review and other means of evaluation to assure the quality of nursing practice. (Reprinted with permission from Standards and Scope of Nursing Practice. Copyright 1987 by the American Nurses' Association, Kansas City, MO.)

LIST OF TABLES

Integumentary Conditions

HERPESVIRUS VARICELLA ZOSTER

After an infection of chicken pox during childhood, the virus becomes dormant within the spinal or cranial dorsal root ganglia. During adulthood, reactivation of the virus may be triggered by a compromised immunologic state, chronic debilitation, acute illness, local trauma, stress, or the presence of lymphomas. Older adults are more likely to suffer from herpes zoster because of their diminishing immunologic response. The rash usually subsides with frequent residual scarring in 10–14 days. However, post-herpetic pain can persist for months or years after the lesions have healed. The incidence of post-herpetic neuralgia (PHN) increases with the age of the patient. It is also more common and lasts longer when the trigeminal nerve is involved.

ETIOLOGIES
- Herpes zoster [varicella zoster virus (VZV)]

CLINICAL MANIFESTATIONS
Herpes zoster begins with
- malaise
- mild aches and pains
- nausea
- chills and fever

followed by
- severe pain, itching, hyperesthesia, and burning along the distribution of a nerve
- unilateral eruption of vesicles
- erythematous plaques progressing to vesicles filled with clear fluid that becomes purulent
- open lesions with seeping and crusting
- fever
- malaise

3

CLINICAL/DIAGNOSTIC FINDINGS
- Visualization of dermatomic distribution of lesions
- Tzanck test of vesicular fluid with eosinophil intranuclear inclusions and varicella virus

---

Clinical Clip

Post-herpetic neuralgia is reported to be the principal cause of intractable, debilitating pain in the elderly and leading cause of suicide in chronic pain sufferers over age 70. About 50% of people who reach 85 years will have had shingles, and most of them will also suffer protracted pain of PHN.

▶ **NURSING DIAGNOSIS:** *Pain*

Related To inflammation of sensory nerves to the skin area.

Defining Characteristics
- Verbalization from patient
- Disorientation
- Withdrawal
- Changes in body posture
- Facial expressions of discomfort

Patient Outcomes
The patient will verbalize relief of pain, itching, and burning.

Nursing Interventions	Rationales
Examine patient to determine cause of pain if diagnosis has not yet been identified.	The pain of herpes zoster often mimics conditions ranging from muscle strain to myocardial infarction. The skin eruptions may not appear until 24–48 h after the onset of pain.
Administer analgesics as prescribed by physician.	Unrelieved pain can lead to anxiety, exhaustion, and depression.

Nursing Interventions	Rationales
Consider alternative pain relief methods such as biofeedback or transcutaneous electrical nerve stimulation (TENS).	Alternative methods may enhance the action of medication.
Administer oral prednisone as prescribed.	Oral prednisone given early in the course of the disease reduces inflammation, thus reducing pain and decreasing the risk of post-herpetic neuralgia.
Administer oral antidepressants as prescribed.	Unrelieved pain can lead to decreased nutritional intake and physical inactivity, both of which can result in other complications including depression.

▶ NURSING DIAGNOSIS: *High Risk for Infection*

Risk Factors
- Impaired skin integrity due to vesicles and lesions
- Compromised immunologic response
- Scratching due to pruritus
- Chronic debilitation

Patient Outcomes
The patient will remain free of complications related to infection.

Nursing Interventions	Rationales
Evaluate patient's medical history and medication regime.	Herpes zoster and resulting complications can be devastating to immunocompromised patients, attacking internal organs. Without treatment, there may be permanent injury, such as paralysis or loss of sight or hearing, or death from viral pneumonia or secondary bacterial infection can occur. At high risk for complications are persons

Nursing Interventions	Rationales
	with acquired immunodeficiency syndrome (AIDS), those taking immunosuppressing drugs after organ transplants, or those taking cortisone and certain anticancer agents.
Monitor for signs and symptoms of headache, weakness, fever, and stiff neck.	It is important to identify and treat central nervous system (CNS) complications which can affect any elderly person with herpes zoster.
Examine body (including the face) thoroughly to detect location of lesions.	The skin lesions are usually confined to a narrow band on one side only. Individual nerve ganglia serve either the left or right side of the body, but not both sides. The lesions may surround one eye and the nose. Lesions on the eyelid are not a threat to the eye itself. A lesion on the tip of the nose means that the cornea will be affected with possible loss of vision in that eye.
Cleanse skin with normal saline. Apply astringent compresses as prescribed and change q8–12h.	Compresses soften and loosen crusts and reduce pruritus, minimizing the tendency to scratch.
Apply topical antimicrobial agents as prescribed.	Antimicrobial agents will prevent the growth of bacteria.
Maintain personal hygiene.	Personal cleanliness reduces the risk of infection.
Instruct to avoid scratching. Clean and trim fingernails regularly.	Scratching impairs skin integrity, allowing for entrance of bacteria from the fingernails.
Provide with soft toothbrush and saline for oral care.	Adequate mouth care and appropriate diet will preclude oral infections.
Advise to eat soft, nutritious, non-irritating foods during acute phase of disease.	Eating appropriate foods prevents injury to the mucous membranes in the mouth while still providing adequate nutrition.

▶ **NURSING DIAGNOSIS:** *Knowledge Deficit (Treatment of Herpes Zoster)*

Related To inexperience and lack of information regarding herpes zoster. (See Patient Teaching, Appendix C, page 345.)

Defining Characteristics
• Verbalization of problem

Patient Outcomes
The patient will verbalize knowledge of herpes zoster to prevent complications and to avoid the transmission of the disease.

Nursing Interventions	Rationales
Instruct patient on measures to avoid infection (see High Risk for Infection).	Infection can lead to life-threatening complications.
Inform patient of signs and symptoms of complications (see High Risk for Infection).	The patient must be able to quickly identify signs and symptoms that require immediate treatment.
Instruct patient on need for preventing the spread of herpes to other people: visitors, staff, and other patients.	The patient should avoid close contact with persons who have not had chicken pox (see Table 1.1, page 8).
Provide information on medications (see Table 1.2, page 8).	Knowledge facilitates compliance.

DISCHARGE PLANNING/CONTINUITY OF CARE
• Verify patient's/family's knowledge of prescribed medications.
• Verify patient's/family's ability to identify signs and symptoms of complications.

Table 1.1 • Isolation Procedures for Herpes Zoster

Immunocompromised Patients or Disseminated Herpes	Private room Masks for susceptible persons Gloves for touching lesion secretions and possibly respiratory secretions Gowns
Localized Herpes in Normal Patient	Private room if hygiene is poor No masks No gowns Gloves for lesion secretions until lesions crusted

Table 1.2 • Medications for Herpes Zoster

Acyclovir Ointment	Apply a $\frac{1}{2}$-in. ribbon of ointment on each 4-in. square of skin Thoroughly cover all lesions Wear glove or finger cot to avoid transmission to other body areas
Prednisone	Avoid sudden stopping of drug Monitor weight, blood pressure, K^+, sleep patterns, blood glucose if diabetic Report delayed wound healing

BIBLIOGRAPHY

Cuzzell, J. Z. (1990). Derm detective: Clues: Pain, burning and itching. *American Journal of Nursing, 90*(7), 15–16.

Needham, J. F. (1993). *Gerontological nursing—a restorative approach.* Albany, NY: Delmar.

Neurological Institute of Neurological Disorders and Stroke (NINDS). (August 1991). *Shingles.* Office of Scientific and Health Reports, NINDS. Bethesda, MD.

$\mathcal{P}$RESSURE ULCERS

$\mathbf{P}$ressure ulcers are localized areas of cellular necrosis that tend to occur from prolonged compression of soft tissue between a bony prominence and a firm surface. Pressure can be induced by the bed, chair, restraints, casts, traction devices, splints, orthoses, and tight clothing. Some of the factors which predispose the elderly to pressure ulcers are related to aging changes. (See Aging, Appendix A, page 337.)

ETIOLOGIES
There are four primary causes of pressure ulcers:
- pressure
- friction
- shearing
- moisture

These causes are a result of
- impaired mobility.
- contractures.
- incontinence causing irritation and maceration of the skin.

Other contributing factors include
- altered nutritional status resulting in inadequate protein/albumin levels.
- predisposing disease processes contributing to a debilitated state.
- altered sensation causing delayed or diminished response to pain and pressure.
- cognitive impairment resulting in unawareness of pressure and immobility.

CLINICAL MANIFESTATIONS

Stage I
- intact, warm , pink, red, or mottled skin

Stage II
- abrasion, blister, shallow crater
- partial thickness ulcer confined to epidermal and/or dermal layers
- surrounding skin red or dusky

Stage III
- full-thickness skin ulcer with deep tissue involvement, may extend to but not through fascia
- exposure of subcutaneous tissue
- exudate usually present
- necrosis may be present
- sinus tracts may be present

Stage IV
- full-thickness skin ulcer with penetration of fascia
- muscle, bone, and supporting structures exposed and destroyed

CLINICAL/DIAGNOSTIC FINDINGS
- Presence of pressure ulcer
- Leukocyte count > 10,000/mm^3 if ulcer is infected
- Total serum protein < 6 g/dL
- Serum albumin < 3.2 g/dL

▶ NURSING DIAGNOSIS: *Impaired Tissue Integrity*

Related To pressure causing capillary occlusion that prevents the flow of blood to and from tissue cells.

Defining Characteristics
- Destroyed integument
- Destroyed subcutaneous tissue

Patient Outcomes
The patient will be free of impaired tissue integrity, as evidenced by
- lack of redness.
- absence of breaks in the integument.
- healed subcutaneous tissue.

Nursing Interventions

Complete pressure ulcer risk assessment (see Table 2.1, page 21), and assess the stage of the existing ulcer.

NOTE: Assess ulcer weekly and measure width, length, and depth to determine progress of treatment (see Table 2.4, page 24).

Rationales

Implementing preventive measures for high-risk patients can prevent further breakdown and facilitate healing of existing ulcers. Treatment is based upon the stage and color of the wound (see Table 2.2, page 22, and Table 2.3, page 24.) Inappropriate treatment may delay healing or precipitate further tissue damage.

Nursing Interventions

Evaluate wound for presence of eschar, indicating a need for debridement. Assess wound for vascular status before debridement is initiated. Prepare for wound debridement:

1. Surgical debridement may be done with or without grafting. The procedure may include
   - local excision.
   - removal of bony prominences.
   - split- or full-thickness grafting.
   - transposition of muscle into ulcerated areas.
   - creation of rotational skin flaps.
2. Mechanical debridement is accomplished with wet-to-damp dressings. This procedure is effective if only limited debridement is needed and there is minimal drainage.
   - Soak 4 × 4-in. gauze dressings in normal saline or lactated Ringer's solution, wring out excess moisture, and apply to wound.
   - Change q3–4h.
3. Chemical debridement requires the use of enzymatic agents. Chemical debridement may be used in conjunction with surgical debridement. Follow manufacturer's instructions for use of enzymatic agents.
4. Autolytic debridement requires occlusive/semiocclusive dressings to create a moist environment.

Cleanse ulcer with normal saline or lactated Ringer's solution when area is soiled and before application of therapy. Minimize the force and friction applied to the skin.

Rationales

Tissue repair cannot begin if the wound is covered with eschar. Adequate blood supply is necessary. Dry ischemic wounds may not have sufficient blood flow to support wound healing. If the eschar is removed, the open wound may become infected. If left dry, the necrotic tissue may become loose without intervention, causing less tissue loss. Debridement methods are selected on the basis of the extent of eschar present: Mechanical debridement is recommended only when limited debridement is needed and there is minimal drainage. During mechanical debridement, dressings should not be allowed to dry. Removal of dry dressings is painful and impedes healing by destroying the fibroblasts from the wound base. Some experts recommend the use of autolytic and chemical debridement only to supplement surgical debridement.

Normal saline is physiologically neutral and nonirritating to healthy tissue. Lactated Ringer's solution contains electrolytes and is conducive to tissue growth. Hydrogen

Nursing Interventions	Rationales
	peroxide, povidone-iodine, acetic acid, and Dakin's solution may be irritating to healthy skin surrounding the wound. These solutions can disturb capillaries in the granulation tissue and are often toxic to fibroblasts. Epithelialization may be impeded and collagen synthesis impaired.
Determine whether healing or maintenance is the goal. 1. Implement therapy selected on the basis of • stage of ulcer. • amount and type of drainage. • presence of dead space. 2. Treatment should meet these criteria: • provide moist environment • provide patient comfort • protect from trauma and infection • be cost effective NOTE: See Tables 2.2 and 2.3, pages 22–24, for summary and selection of treatments.	Healing may not always be achievable if the patient is dying or has dry, uninfected ulcers related to peripheral vascular disease. To support healing, maintain a balance between absorption of excessive exudate and a moist environment. The moist environment encourages autolytic debridement, allowing white blood cells to break down eschar and slough. Cost must be considered as reimbursement of wound care supplies by Medicare and Medicaid varies between states and may also depend on the location of care (hospital, long-term care facility, or home).
Instruct/demonstrate to caregiver and have caregiver return demonstration for 1. cleansing and application of therapy if patient is returning home. 2. proper disposal of soiled supplies.	The predisposing factors for the pressure ulcer (impaired mobility) are likely to prevent the patient from caring for the ulcer. A home health care nurse may not be available for every application.

▶ **NURSING DIAGNOSIS:** *Impaired Physical Mobility*

Related To
• Lack of endurance or strength
• Neuromuscular or musculoskeletal disease
• Activity intolerance

- Pain with movement
- Depression

Defining Characteristics
- Limited range of motion (ROM)
- Impaired coordination and balance
- Reluctance to move
- Loss of muscle strength and mass
- Easily fatigued

Patient Outcomes
The patient will
- be relieved of pressure over bony prominences.
- remain free of contractures.

The patient or caregiver will
- verbalize understanding of the necessity for mobility.
- demonstrate pressure-relieving techniques.

Nursing Interventions	Rationales
Institute pressure-relieving measures: 1. Establish schedule and change position at least q2h or more often. 2. Place pressure-relieving devices in bed and chair. 3. Teach pressure-relieving wheelchair exercises. 4. Check areas of potential pressure under casts and orthotic and prosthetic devices frequently. 5. Avoid the use of restraints.	The effectiveness of any treatment is obliterated if pressure is not relieved. Healing cannot take place without adequate blood flow to the area. Pressure > 35 mm Hg for 1–2 h may cause ischemia. Sitting exerts more pressure on the coccyx and gluteal muscles than does lying in bed. Teaching weight-shifting exercises while sitting relieves this pressure. The use of restraints inhibits mobility and may cause pressure and friction if not applied properly.
Institute measures to avoid friction and shearing of the skin: 1. Use turning sheet to move patient in bed or chair. 2. Use appropriate transfer techniques. 3. Avoid the use of powder on the patient's skin. 4. Place bed cradle under top covers.	Friction occurs when two surfaces move across each other, causing disruption of epithelial cells and accelerating the process of ulceration. This occurs when the skin of the buttocks rubs across the bed as the patient is moved without a turning sheet, when the patient is dragged off of or onto the bed during an inappropriate transfer,

Nursing Interventions	Rationales
5. Keep head of bed lower than 30° unless contraindicated. 6. Use supportive devices to prevent sliding in chairs.	and when the bed covers rub on the patient's toes. Powder on the skin acts as an abrasive as it mixes with body moisture and causes beading. Shearing occurs when layers of tissue slide on each other. The superficial fascia slides, but the sacral skin remains stationary due to the friction from the sheets. The subcutaneous blood vessels are twisted and distorted, preventing blood flow. This occurs when the patient slides down in the bed or in the chair.
Prevent spasticity and contracture formation: 1. Avoid quick, rough movements. 2. Do ROM exercises at least twice daily. 3. Administer antispasmodics if prescribed.	Contractures develop more readily in the presence of spasticity and often precede formation of pressure ulcers. A contracture increases the pressure of the joint against the mattress or chair, further impeding circulation. Spasticity may be avoided when extremities are handled in a gentle, smooth manner. Doing ROM exercises with each motion five to seven times twice a day can prevent the onset of contractures.
Instruct/demonstrate to caregiver/patient and have caregiver/patient return demonstrations for correct techniques for positioning, transfers, and ROM exercises. Instruct patient in techniques for self-mobility in bed, if not contraindicated.	Healing will not occur unless mobility program is continued.

▶ **NURSING DIAGNOSIS:** *Altered Urinary Elimination*

Related To
- Sensory motor impairment
- Urinary tract infection
- Ineffective detrusor muscle

Defining Characteristics
• Incontinence

Patient Outcomes
The patient will remain clean and dry.

Nursing Interventions	Rationales
Prevent moisture buildup and maintain skin cleanliness: 1. Implement bladder management program (see Incontinence, page 165). 2. Use absorbent incontinent briefs or pads if other bladder management programs fail. 3. Check for incontinence frequently. Wash, rinse, and dry perirectal area thoroughly and apply moisture barrier. Use a mild cleansing agent, avoid hot water, and use minimal force and friction during the cleaning process. 4. Avoid use of plastic/rubber sheets and protectors.	Perspiration, urine, and feces are skin irritants that change the pH of the skin, supporting growth of skin flora and increasing the possibility of infection. Incontinent briefs/pads have a wicking action, preventing moisture buildup on the skin. Using care during the cleaning process avoids further destruction to frail skin. Plastic and rubber trap moisture and produce heat, further facilitating skin breakdown.
Instruct caregiver/patient and ask for verbalization of understanding in 1. the selected bladder management procedures. 2. cleansing techniques.	Ongoing care is essential to avoid continuing skin and tissue impairment.

▶ NURSING DIAGNOSIS: *Altered Nutrition—Less than Body Requirements*

Related To biological, economical, or psychosocial factors causing difficulty with ingestion or digestion of nutrients.

Defining Characteristics
Weight loss without conscious calorie restrictions:
• Five percent weight loss in 1 month is considered significant, >5% is severe.
• Over a 3-month period 7.5% loss is significant, >7.5% is severe.

- Over a 6-month period 10% loss is significant, >10% is severe.

Laboratory values:
- hemoglobin (Hgb) <14 g/dL in men, <12 g/dL in women
- hematocrit (Hct) <40% men, <37% in women
- total iron-binding capacity (TIBC) >420 µg/dL
- total protein <6 g/dL
- serum albumin <3.2 g/dL
- serum globulin <2.3 g/dL

Patient Outcomes

The patient will
- consume 75% or more from each food group served at each meal.
- attain or maintain body weight in accordance with age, body structure, and height.
- attain laboratory values within the accepted range:
  –Hgb: men, 14–18 g/dL; women, 12–16 g/dL
  –Hct: men, 42–52%; women, 37–47%
  –TIBC: 250–420 µg/dL
  –total protein: 6–8 g/dL
  –serum albumin: 3.2–4.5 g/dL
  –serum globulin: 2.3–3.4 g/dL
- maintain daily fluid intake of 1,500–2,000 mL unless contraindicated.

Nursing Interventions	Rationales
Assess nutritional status: 1. anthropometric measurements • height and weight • triceps skin fold (TSF) • midarm circumference (MAC) • midarm muscle circumference (MAMC) 2. laboratory studies	The use of anthropometric measurements for evaluating body composition in the elderly is useful when considered with the other assessment data. Triceps skin fold estimates the amount of subcutaneous body fat and is useful in predicting pressure ulcer risk. Midarm circumference is an index of the arm's total area and is used to calculate the MAMC, which correlates with total body muscle mass and reflects the caloric adequacy of the patient's previous diet.
Investigate causes of reduced food intake that may be related to the disease process, to aging changes, or to the environment. Assess for	The desire to eat arises from interpretation of sensory stimuli, an intact neural mechanism in the hypothalamus, and an awareness

Nursing Interventions

1. sensory deficits:
   - olfactory
   - gustatory
   - visual
2. cognitive impairment:
   - unaware of hunger
   - inability to attend to eating due to disorientation
   - memory loss
   - short attention span
3. perceptual deficits:
   - agnosia
   - apraxia
   - perseveration
   - latency
   - figure-ground deficits
   - hemianopsia (see Cerebral Vascular Accident, page 224).
4. mobility impairment of upper extremities: inability to bring food to mouth
5. physical discomfort:
   - incorrect positioning
   - pain
   - incontinence
6. chewing problems:
   - poorly fitting dentures
   - edentulous
   - inadequate oral care
7. impaired swallowing (see Enteral Feeding, page 145).
8. anxiety related to physical environment:
   - noise
   - offensive odors
   - inadequate lighting
   - incompatible roommates or table mates
9. ethnic/cultural/religious food choices that differ from the food served.

Rationales

of feelings of hunger. Perceptual deficits may result in inability to see the food or to understand how to get the food to the mouth. Physical dexterity is needed to get the food to the mouth for chewing and swallowing.

Nursing Interventions	Rationales
Correct underlying nutritional deficits: 1. Study assessment data to formulate interventions. 2. Request swallowing assessment, if indicated, from speech pathologist or occupational therapist. 3. Request assessment of perceptual deficits from occupational therapist if necessary. 4. Give high-protein supplement if necessary to maintain intake of 45–55 g daily, or more if wound is draining. 5. Increase fluid intake to 2,500–3,000 mL daily unless contraindicated.	Adequate nutrition is required to support wound healing. Adults need 45–55 g of protein daily or 0.6 g/kg of body weight. It is estimated that a draining pressure ulcer loses 30 g of protein daily. Dehydration causes a decrease in blood volume and an increase in blood viscosity. This impedes tissue perfusion.
Monitor weight weekly at the same time of day, on the same scale, and with the same type of clothing.	Obtaining weekly weights provides objective documentation of nutritional intake. Loss of weight can be acted upon immediately.
Instruct patient/caregiver and ask for verbalization of understanding for the 1. need for adequate nutrition. 2. availability of nutritional supplements. 3. procedures for weighing and documentation of weights.	Understanding facilitates compliance.

▶ **NURSING DIAGNOSIS:** *High Risk for Infection*

Risk Factors
- Impaired skin integrity
- Underlying tissue destruction
- Altered nutritional status
- Chronic disease process

Patient Outcomes
The patient will remain free of infection.

Nursing Interventions	Rationales
Implement use of universal precautions for all patients. Utilize sterile treatment procedures in the hospital and long-term care facility. Clean technique rather than sterile may be appropriate in the home setting.	The threat of nosocomial infection is nonexistent in the home. It is difficult to maintain completely sterile technique in the home.
Monitor for clinical signs of infection: 1. elevated temperature (>38 C) 2. heat 3. redness 4. localized swelling 5. localized tenderness or pain 6. purulent drainage 7. elevated leukocyte count 8. mental status changes **NOTE:** Elderly persons do not present with signs and symptoms 1–7 as readily as younger persons due to changes in the immunologic system. Mental status changes may be an early indicator of infection.	All pressure ulcers are colonized with bacteria, but not all are infected. Signs of local inflammation and drainage are the most important indicators of infection. Complications such as cellulitis, osteomyelitis, bacteremia, and sepsis can develop quickly, causing serious illness and even death.
Collect drainage specimen for culture and sensitivity if clinical signs are present.	Pressure ulcer infections are usually polymicrobial. The incidence of colonization or infection with antibiotic-resistant organisms is higher in nursing home patients. Accurate collection of pretreatment cultures permits correct antibiotic treatment.
Use correct technique to collect wound culture: 1. Irrigate with sterile normal saline (not antiseptic solution) and debride surface, if necessary, of loose necrotic substance. Use sterile gauze pad to absorb saline.	Using an antiseptic solution can kill the causative microorganism. Cleansing removes external exudate which, if cultured, will not give the true cause of the underlying infection. Cleansing also removes antibiotic ointments. An accurate culture is more likely if it is obtained from viable tissue.

Nursing Interventions	Rationales
2. Collect specimen from clean and viable granulation tissue using swabs from prepackaged culture tube. Place specimen in prepackaged culture tube containing transport medium. Send to laboratory within 1–2 h.	Using a prepackaged culture tube assures sterility of the swabs. Transporting the specimen immediately in the right medium avoids death of the microorganisms.
Instruct caregiver and request verbalization of knowledge for 1. measures for prevention of infection. 2. signs of clinical infection. 3. notification of appropriate health care professional (physician or home health nurse) if signs of infection are present (see Appendix C, page 345).	Preventive measures are mandatory due to the high risk for infection when skin integrity is impaired. Prompt identification of signs of infection permits prompt treatment.

DISCHARGE PLANNING/CONTINUITY OF CARE

- Arrange for home-delivered meals if necessary.
- Arrange for home health nurse to provide on-going evaluation, to implement therapy, and to continue the instruction.
- Arrange with durable medical equipment supplier to provide pressure-relieving devices.
- Inform patient/family where dressing supplies can be purchased.
- Provide information on payment sources (if available) for services, supplies, and equipment.
- Conduct home assessment for environmental safety (see Safety Assessment, Appendix B, page 343).

--- Clinical Clip ---

Five to 10% of hospitalized patients suffer skin breakdown; $3.5 billion to $7 billion are spent annually to prevent or heal pressure ulcers. The cost of nursing time increases 50%, and the cost of treatment is $10,000–$15,000 per ulcer.

Table 2.1 • Pressure Ulcer Risk Assessment

Name _____ Adm. No._____

Date _____ Pressure ulcer present on admission?_____

		Total
Activity		
Ambulant without assistance	0	
Ambulant with assistance	2	
Chairfast	4	
Bedfast	6	_____
Mobility		
Full ROM	0	
Moves with minimal assistance	2	
Moves with moderate assistance	4	
Immobile	6	_____
Skin condition		
Hydrated and intact	0	
Rashes or abrasions	2	
Decreased turgor, dry	4	
Edema, erythema, pressure ulcers	6	_____
Predisposing disease process		
No involvement	0	
Chronic, stable	1	
Acute or chronic, unstable	2	
Terminal	3	_____
Level of consciousness		
Alert	0	
Slow verbal response	1	
Responds to verbal or painful stimuli	2	
Absence of response to stimuli	3	_____
Nutritional status		
Eats 75% or more of required intake	0	
Eats less than 75%	1	
Minimal intake, consistent weight loss	2	
Unable/refuses to eat/drink, emaciated	3	_____

Table 2.1 • *continued*

Incontinence—bladder		
None	0	
Less than 2 times over 24 h	1	
More than 2 times over 24 h	2	
Total, no control	3	_____
Incontinence—bowel		
None	0	
Occasional, formed stool	1	
Usually, semiformed stool	2	
Total, no control, loose stool	3	_____
	Total score	_____

Score of 11–20: moderate risk. Score of 21–23: high risk.

Source: Adapted from "Skin Care of Older Adults" by Fowler, E., 1985, Journal of Gerontological Nursing, 11*(11), p. 44. Copyright 1982. Reprinted by permission.*

Table 2.2 • Summary of Treatments

1. Transparent, thin-film, semipermeable, semiocclusive dressings: for Stages II and III with minimal drainage; may liquefy black eschar or necrotic tissue; contraindicated for infected wounds

   - Allow for exchange of oxygen and moisture vapor
   - Do not allow passage of fluid or bacteria
   - Exudate forms from white blood cells and serum, bathing wound and providing moist environment
   - Transparency allows easy visualization
   - Can be left in place up to 7 days unless there are signs of leakage, infection, or maceration
   - Available with pouches for wounds with larger amounts of drainage

2. Hydrocolloid collusive wafers: for Stage II and III wounds and other superficial wounds with moderate exudate; contraindicated for infected wounds or when bone or tendon is visible; debride black eschar and necrotic tissue before application

   - Hydroactive and absorptive particles interact with wound exudate to form a gel, creating a moist environment that promotes healing

Table 2.2 • *continued*

- Protects new tissue
- Provides moderate absorption and moist wound surface
- Necrotic tissue liquified by autolysis
- Prevents entry of bacteria to wound
- Helps prevent shearing
- May be left in place for up to 1 week; change when saturated or when leakage or separation occurs

3. Gel dressings
- Occlusive if plastic backing left on one side; semiocclusive if backing removed from both sides
- Some brands may require additional occlusive dressing
- Moist, soothing, moderately absorptive, and nonadhesive
- Require frequent reapplication to avoid dehydration of gel

4. Polyurethane foam
- Semipermeable, do not adhere to wound or surrounding skin
- Surface is hydrophobic
- Maintain moisture

5. Dextranomers: absorption beads, flakes, granules
- Use only on draining wounds
- Reduce edema
- Absorb exudate, bacteria, odor

6. Calcium alginate dressings
- For wounds with exudate
- Gel forms when dressing comes in contact with wound
- Normal saline irrigation required before application
- Secondary dressing required
- May need frequent changes due to large amounts of exudate

Table 2.3 • The Three-Color Concept for Treatment Selection

Assess the color of open wounds healing by secondary intention to select the appropriate treatment:

1. **Red wounds:** granulation tissue covers wound bed, becoming beefy red as the layer thickens

   Treatment: Keep clean, moist; protect from trauma

2. **Yellow wounds:** exudate is white with yellow tinge, creamy yellow, ivory, or yellowish green

   Treatment: Irrigate to remove exudate, keep wound moist

3. **Black wounds:** necrotic, avascular tissue

   Treatment: Debride, keep wound moist

Table 2.4 • Documentation of Pressure Ulcer Healing and Treatment

Document at least weekly:

- Date
- Site of pressure ulcer
- Stage of pressure ulcer
- Size: length, width, depth
- Color
- Odor
- Drainage (describe)
- Tunneling
- Inflammation

BIBLIOGRAPHY

Agency for Health Care Policy and Research. (1992). *Clinical Practice Guideline Number 3. Pressure ulcers in adults: Prediction and prevention.* Rockville, MD: U.S. Department of Health and Human Services.

Barnes, H. R. (1993a). Alternating transparent and hydrocolloid dressings. *Nursing 93, 23*(3), 59–61.

Barnes, H. R. (1993b). Wound care: Facts and fiction about hydrocolloid dressings. *Journal of Gerontological Nursing, 19*(6), 23–26.

Brown-Etris, M., Arnold, N., & Russ, G. (1993). The wound care puzzle. *Ostomy/Wound Management, 39*(2); 45–46, 50–54, 56, 59–60.

Burd, C., Langemo, D. K., Olson, B., Hanson, D., Hunter, S., & Sauvage, T. (1992). Skin problems: Epidemiology of pressure ulcers in a skilled care facility. *Journal of Gerontological Nursing, 18*(9), 29–39.

Cuzzell, J. A. (1993). The right way to culture a wound. *American Journal of Nursing, 93*(5), 48–50.

Jahnigen, D. W. (1992). Infectious complications of pressure ulcers. *Geriatric Focus on Infectious Diseases, 2*(5), 1–3, 12.

Krainski, M. (1992). Pressure ulcers and the elderly. *Ostomy/Wound Management, 38*(5), 22, 24, 26.

Krasner, D. (1992). Resolving the dressing dilemma: Selecting wound dressing by category. *Plastic Surgical Nursing, 12*(1), 22–27.

Needham, J. F. (1993). *Gerontological nursing—a restorative approach.* Albany, NY: Delmar.

Resnick, B. (1993). Wound care for the elderly. *Geriatric Nursing, 14*(1), 26–29.

Smith, P. W. (1992). Approach to nursing home patients with skin and soft tissue infections. In R. J. Duma (Ed.), *Recognition and management of nursing home infections.* Bethesda, MD: National Foundation for Infectious Diseases.

Thomas-Hess, C. (1992). Pressure ulcers—current treatment trends. *Nursing Homes, 41*(5), 37–40.

Thomas-Hess, C. (1993). Pressure ulcers: Keys to prevention. *Nursing Homes, 42*(4), 31–32.

$\mathcal{S}$CABIES

$\mathcal{S}$cabies is a highly infectious skin disease which can be easily transmitted among the elderly in long-term care facilities. Poor hygiene and crowded conditions increase the risk for acquiring the disease. Scabies is transmitted by direct contact through the skin or sexual relations. It takes 4–6 weeks from contact to emergence of symptoms. Persons previously infected develop symptoms within 1–4 days after reexposure.

ETIOLOGIES
- *Sarcoptes scabiei* var. *hominis* (itch mite): transmission is direct skin-to-skin contact.

CLINICAL MANIFESTATIONS
NOTE: The incubation period for scabies is 4–6 weeks. The initial stages of the disease cause few or no signs and symptoms.

- Red rash with linear burrows appearing between the fingers and on the extensor surface of elbows, hands, flexor surface of wrists, axillary folds, waistline, creases of buttocks, nipples in females, and genitalia in males
- Grayish-white thread on surface of skin, marking trail of female mite
- Itching that increases at night

CLINICAL/DIAGNOSTIC FINDINGS
- Observance of characteristic trails
- Superficial skin scraping examined under low-power microscope (choose lesions which have not been excoriated by scratching)

▶ NURSING DIAGNOSIS: *High Risk for Impaired Skin Integrity*

Risk Factors
- Penetration of female mite into epidermis for egg-laying creating a microscopic opening in the epidermis

- Scratching of skin due to itching

Patient Outcomes
The patient will be free of skin impairments and consequent risk of infection.

Nursing Interventions	Rationales
Try to identify the source of the scabies. In a long-term care facility, consider application of scabicide to all residents as a preventive measure. Apply scabicide (wear gown and gloves) according to manufacturer's directions: 1. Wash entire body with soap and water. 2. Apply thin layer of cream from neck down. Give special attention to folds, creases, interdigital spaces, area around nails, and genital area. 3. Do not apply to face, eyes, or mucous membranes. 4. Wash off after 12–48 h according to manufacturer's directions. Apply second coat if recommended.	Applying scabicide to all patients in long-term care facilities will cure cases that may not have been yet diagnosed. Scabicides will be effective only if applied correctly.
Reassure that itching will cease, although it may continue for 2–3 weeks after treatment. Monitor for signs of irritation or hypersensitivity. Wash off and notify physician. Monitor for new lesions and need for retreatment.	Scabicide exterminates the mites and the eggs, curing the disease within 12–48 h, although itching may persist. There are few adverse reactions to most scabicides. However, manifestations of such need to be treated promptly.

▶ NURSING DIAGNOSIS: *Sleep Pattern Disturbance*
Related To pruritus that increases at night.

Defining Characteristics
- Complaints of patient
- Observations of frequent wakefulness

Patient Outcomes

The patient will
- experience longer sleep periods.
- verbalize feeling of restfulness.

Nursing Interventions	Rationales
Apply antipruritic emollient or topical steroid after treatment if prescribed.	Reducing pruritus decreases the desire to scratch.
Administer oral antihistamine if prescribed.	Oral antihistamines reduce pruritus.
Consider distraction techniques.	Lack of sleep can affect older adults' ability to function adequately and can lead to disorientation. Distraction techniques may be effective.

▶ NURSING DIAGNOSIS: *Altered Health Maintenance*

Related To
- Perceptual/cognitive deficits
- Impaired mobility
- Ineffective coping

Defining Characteristics
- Inadequate gross or fine motor skills required to maintain activities of daily living (ADL)
- Demonstrated lack of knowledge regarding personal hygiene

Patient Outcomes

The patient will maintain (with assistance if necessary) adequate personal hygiene.

Nursing Interventions	Rationales
Assess abilities to complete ADL.	Patient may require community health care services if living at home.

Nursing Interventions	Rationales
Place patients in hospitals or long-term care facilities in wound and skin precautions until 24 h after effective treatment.	Scabies is highly contagious.
Sterilize all clothing and bed linens after treatment is completed. Repeat if retreatment is required.	Sterilization avoids reinfection of patient.
Take precautions to avoid the accidental exchanging of clothing, bed linens, and towels in hospitals and long-term care facilities. Instruct to wash hands often, shampoo hair frequently, and wear clean clothes every day.	It is questionable whether scabies can be transmitted through clothing, linens, and towels, but this precaution is usually implemented in group living facilities.

DISCHARGE PLANNING/CONTINUITY OF CARE
- Reinforce need for adequate personal hygiene.
- Arrange for homemaker or home health aide if patient is unable to adequately care for self and environment.
- Instruct patient/caregiver to observe for signs of recurring infestation.
- Conduct home assessment for environmental safety (see Safety Assessment, Appendix B, page 343).

Clinical Clip

In elderly and immunodeficient patients, the infestation may appear as a generalized dermatitis with scaling, vesiculation, and crusting (Norwegian scabies). Itching may be diminished or absent. This form is highly contagious and may be present for a period of time before diagnosis is made. It is commonly seen in the chronically ill.

BIBLIOGRAPHY
Benensom, A. S., & Legters, L. J. (1990). *Communicable diseases*. Washington, DC: American Public Health Association.

Hench, C., Paulson, S. S., Stevens, D. A., & Thompson, J. D. (1994). Scabies outbreak on a spinal cord injury unit. *Rehabilitation Nursing, 19*(1), 21–23.

Needham, J. F. (1993). *Gerontological nursing—a restorative approach*. Albany, NY: Delmar.

$\mathcal{S}$KIN CANCER

The incidence of cancer, including that of the skin, increases with age. There are four major types of skin cancer: basal cell carcinoma, squamous cell carcinoma, melanoma, and Kaposi's sarcoma.

ETIOLOGIES

The primary risk factor for basal cell carcinoma, squamous cell carcinoma, and melanoma is exposure to ultraviolet light. Kaposi's sarcoma is seen in patients with acquired immunodeficiency syndrome (AIDS) or in renal transplant patients receiving immunosuppressive drugs.

CLINICAL MANIFESTATIONS

- Basal cell
  - Flesh-colored or pink translucent nodule with superimposed telangiectasis
  - Ulceration may accompany growth of the tumor
  - Tumor can grow over a period of years and metastasize, destroying facial structures
- Squamous cell
  - Reddish color
  - Plaques that may be ulcerated or covered with crust
- Melanoma
  - Color variation
  - Asymmetrical
  - Irregular border
  - Diameter > 6 mm
- Kaposi's sarcoma
  - Lymphadenopathy
  - Weight loss
  - Diarrhea
  - Fatigue
  - Dark-blue to reddish-purple nodules or spots on arms and legs

CLINICAL/DIAGNOSTIC FINDINGS

Biopsy of the lesion indicates the presence of malignant cells.

▶ NURSING DIAGNOSIS: *Fear*

Related To perceptions of death resulting from cancer.

Defining Characteristics
- Verbalization of concerns
- Increased tension
- Inability to function adequately due to apprehension

Patient Outcomes
The patient will
- verbalize knowledge of the situation.
- demonstrate use of effective coping skills.

Nursing Interventions	Rationales
Actively listen to concerns.	Verbalization reduces tension.
Provide information regarding treatment in verbal and written form. (See Patient Teaching, Appendix C, page 345.)	Receiving factual information decreases the apprehension related to the "unknown."
Determine effective coping skills that have been utilized in past.	The use of previous coping skills may be effective for this situation.
Observe interactions with significant other(s).	Intervention may be necessary if significant others are reinforcing the fears of the patient. If the significant others are supportive, they can assist the patient to cope with the situation.
Provide information and access to local cancer support groups.	Support groups can ease the patient's fears and provide emotional comfort.

▶ NURSING DIAGNOSIS: *Altered Nutrition—Less Than Body Requirements*

Related To inability to ingest food due to effects of treatment (radiation or chemotherapy)

NOTE: Basal cell and squamous cell carcinoma are generally surgically excised. Radiation and/or chemotherapy may be implemented for melanoma and Kaposi's sarcoma.

Defining Characteristics
- Observance of inadequate food intake
- Loss of weight
- Reported altered taste sensation

Patient Outcomes
The patient will
- maintain usual weight.
- maintain adequate nutritional status.

Nursing Interventions	Rationales
Administer prophylactic therapy before and after treatment as prescribed.	Prophylactic therapy reduces the risk of nausea and vomiting.
Consider the use of relaxation therapy, distraction techniques, or guided imagery.	These techniques augment the use of medication in the control of nausea and vomiting.
Arrange for tolerable foods and pleasant dining environment: 1. Give dry, bland foods before meals. 2. Give small, frequent, high-caloric-density foods. 3. Create relaxed, pleasant eating atmosphere. 4. Experiment with seasonings and varied food combinations. 5. Avoid offensive foods and minimize food odors. 6. Advise to eat and drink slowly.	Maintaining adequate nutritional status is essential. Interventions may be needed to reduce nausea associated with eating and anxiety due to the food or the environment.

▶ NURSING DIAGNOSIS: *High Risk for Infection*

Risk Factors
- Cancer treatments
- Altered nutrition
- Underlying disease process

Patient Outcomes
The patient will be free of infections.

Nursing Interventions	Rationales
Monitor for signs of infection: 1. fever 2. lethargy 3. subtle changes in vital signs 4. irritability 5. confusion	Promptly identifying infection allows for prompt treatment.
Implement pressure ulcer prevention program.	Impaired skin integrity due to pressure ulcer increases the risk of infection.
Change position frequently; encourage to cough and deep breathe.	These interventions reduce the risk of respiratory infections.
Administer stool softeners if necessary.	Constipation increases the risk of infection.
Provide mouth care around the clock.	Avoid impairment of mucous membranes.
Implement universal precautions.	Avoid nosocomial infections associated with cross contamination.

▶ **NURSING DIAGNOSIS:** *Knowledge Deficit (Cancer Prevention and Warning Signs)*

Related To lack of information regarding cancer prevention (see Appendix C, page 345).

Defining Characteristics
• Verbalization of problem
• Requests for information

Patient Outcomes
The patient will
• verbalize knowledge of cancer prevention methods.
• verbalize knowledge of the signs of cancer.
• demonstrate skin self-examination.

Nursing Interventions	**Rationales**
Teach technique for monthly skin self-exam: 1. Examine the skin once a month after the shower or bath. 2. Make sure the room is well-lit and the necessary items are available: • full-length mirror • hand-held mirror • hand-held blow dryer • two chairs or stools	There is a risk of reoccurrence of skin cancer. A monthly skin self-exam leads to early treatment and increases the chance for cure.
Provide for instruction of nursing assistants in long-term care facilities and family members or the home health aide in home care.	The procedure may be difficult for elderly individuals with impaired vision and diminished joint flexibility.
Provide information on prevention guidelines: 1. Minimize sun exposure and avoid when sun is the strongest. 2. Apply a sunscreen with an SPF (sun protection factor) of at least 15, daily. 3. Wear a hat and cover extremities when out in the sun. 4. Avoid tanning parlors or booths.	Preventive measures will decrease the risk of reoccurrence. Ultraviolet rays are a known carcinogen. Avoiding exposure to carcinogens reduces the risk of skin cancer.

DISCHARGE PLANNING/CONTINUITY OF CARE
- Provide instructions for continuing treatments if necessary.
- Verify patient's/family's knowledge of preventive measures.
- Reinforce instruction on prevention of infection.
- Reinforce need for monthly skin self-exams.

Clinical Clip

- Senile or actinic keratosis is a precancerous growth noted on sun-exposed areas. It presents as a superficial patch covered by a persistent scale.

- Skin cancers are the most common malignancies seen in elderly people. Basal cell carcinoma is the most common, followed by squamous cell carcinoma and malignant melanoma.

BIBLIOGRAPHY

Holleg, A. I., Fink, D. J., & Murphy, G. P. (1991). *Clinical oncology.* Atlanta, GA: American Cancer Society.

Maguire, A. M. (1991). *Skin cancers. A cancer source book for nurses.* Atlanta, GA: American Cancer Society.

Smoller, J., & Smoller, B. R. (1992). Skin malignancies in the elderly. *Journal of Gerontological Nursing, 18*(5), 19–24.

Musculoskeletal Conditions

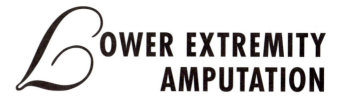

LOWER EXTREMITY AMPUTATION

Insufficient tissue perfusion due to peripheral vascular disease is the most common reason for amputation among elderly patients. Surgery often follows a long period of unsuccessful treatment and discomfort. The patient may or may not be fitted for a prosthetic device. The decision should be made by the patient in consultation with the physician after a thorough evaluation. In any case, the residual limb is always treated as though a prosthesis will be worn. Family/caregiver support is essential for successful rehabilitation.

ETIOLOGIES
- Diabetes
- Trauma
- Circulatory disturbances
- Malignant tumors
- Long-standing bone infections
- Thermal injuries

CLINICAL MANIFESTATIONS
(See Peripheral Vascular Disease, page 97)
Other manifestations dependent upon the reason for the surgery

CLINICAL/DIAGNOSTIC FINDINGS
Dependent upon the reason for the surgery

▶ NURSING DIAGNOSIS: *Knowledge Deficit (Surgical Preparation and Procedure)*

Related To impending surgical removal of limb.

Defining Characteristics
• Verbalization and signs of anxiety related to lack of knowledge

Patient Outcomes
The patient will verbalize knowledge of preoperative and postoperative care.

Nursing Interventions	Rationales
Instruct patient regarding preoperative routine of hospital: 1. nursing assessment and history 2. preoperative diagnostic tests 3. dietary restrictions 4. skin preparation 5. medications 6. monitoring devices and special procedures 7. consent forms	Knowledge facilitates compliance and reduces anxiety.
Instruct patient regarding postoperative care: 1. pain management: postoperative and phantom sensations 2. coughing, turning, and deep breathing 3. dietary management 4. activity level 5. special treatments such as indwelling catheters, intravenous feedings 6. monitoring devices	Patients prepared about the possibility of phantom sensations experience more successful outcomes if the sensations occur.

▶ NURSING DIAGNOSIS: *Pain*

Related To surgery and phantom sensations due to loss of a body part.

Defining Characteristics
• Verbalization of pain
• Distracted behavior
• Facial mask of pain
• Alterations in muscle tone

Patient Outcomes

The patient will

- verbalize relief from surgical pain.
- demonstrate techniques to effectively manage phantom sensations.

Nursing Interventions	Rationales
Assess frequently for pain: patient's perceptions, behavioral responses, and mental status.	Elderly patients are at risk for undertreatment of pain because they may believe it cannot be relieved and therefore do not report pain.
If patient can do so, ask patient to describe severity of pain using a rating scale with 0 as no pain to 10 as the worst possible pain.	The use of rating scales may not be effective if the patient is cognitively impaired. Increased confusion and agitation may be the only indication of pain. Some theories of aging propose that pain tolerance increases with age, but this is not always true. Health care professionals may wrongly believe that pain is a natural consequence of aging. The patient's description is the most reliable indicator of the existence and severity of the pain. Different interventions may be implemented for varying degrees of pain.
Assess other current medical conditions and medication regime.	Pain from other conditions such as arthritis may be extenuating the surgical pain. Medical conditions causing hepatic or renal impairment may cause drug accumulation as most analgesics are metabolized by the liver or kidneys. Pain medication may produce a drug interaction if patient is receiving central nervous system depressants, phenytoin, alcohol, or monoamine oxidase inhibitors. The glomerular filtration rate declines with aging; this can delay the metabolite excretion of opiates, resulting in narcosis and respiratory depression.

Nursing Interventions	Rationales
Administer pain medication as prescribed. Offer medication regularly, before dressing changes, and whenever it is anticipated that pain may be experienced.	Pain that is established and severe is difficult to alleviate. Unrelieved pain has physical and psychological negative consequences and may impede recovery.
Acknowledge presence of phantom sensations and assure that feeling does exist.	The patient may think he or she is psychotic and is hallucinating. The resulting fear and anxiety will increase the phantom sensations and the surgical pain. These sensations do not usually occur until several days or weeks postoperatively and tend to subside within several months. Some amputees report persistent, severe pain for several years. Individuals who experience pain before surgery tend to experience this sensation more often than those who lose a limb suddenly as a result of trauma.
Treat the phantom sensations: 1. Teach relaxation techniques and guided imagery or provide diversional activities. 2. Use counterirritation: cold, warmth, rubbing, pressure.	Learning to control the sensation is a part of the healing process. Medication is not usually effective. Counterirritation works by using a painful stimulus to relieve another painful stimulus.

▶ **NURSING DIAGNOSIS:** *High Risk for Infection*

Risk Factors
- Advanced age
- Underlying problem/impaired circulation
- Fragility of skin
- Decreased immune response

Patient Outcomes
The patient will remain free of infection.

Nursing Interventions	Rationales
Inspect incision area for the following: 1. inflammation 2. breaks in skin 3. drainage 4. edema 5. increased pain 6. hypersensitivity to touch	Prompt assessment of infection indicates prompt treatment, preventing further complications.
Change dressing after each washing of the residual limb and more frequently if drainage is present. Avoid tape. For incontinent patients, cover area with plastic.	Tape causes excoriation. Incontinence contaminates the surgical site.
Instruct patient in care of the residual limb when psychologically ready to participate in care and after sutures are removed (see Patient Teaching, Appendix C, page 345).	Learning will not take place if patient is not mentally ready to learn. The patient's ability to look at the residual limb during care is a good indicator of readiness.
Instruct patient to wash residual limb twice a day with warm water and mild soap. Avoid soaking. Rinse area thoroughly to remove all traces of soap and then pat dry with a clean towel. Air dry the residual limb for 30–40 min before wrapping.	Soaking can increase edema and cause skin maceration, increasing the risk for infection. Soap causes irritation if not thoroughly removed. Air drying prevents maceration.
Instruct patient to avoid the use of ointments, lotions, or other emollients on the surgical site.	These products increase the risk of infection and can cause maceration.
Advise patient to inspect other leg at the same time the residual limb is examined. The remaining leg must be protected against trauma, pressure, or temperature extremes. Cleanliness and a well-fitting shoe and sock are essential.	The remaining leg is at risk for amputation if the underlying etiology was a circulatory disturbance.
Teach patient to prepare the limb for the prosthesis: massage area or brush gently with a washcloth for 3 or 4 min three times a day.	The risk of infection related to skin breakdown from the prosthesis is decreased. Massaging lessens the tenderness and improves vascularity. Brushing toughens the skin.

Nursing Interventions	Rationales
Instruct patient in use of stump socks to be worn with prosthesis. As the residual limb shrinks with the use of the prosthesis, the number of socks or the weight of the socks will need to be increased. If there is swelling, the weight of the socks is decreased. Advise patient to change socks daily and to wash with warm water and mild soap, rinse well, and air dry.	The socks increase comfort with the prosthesis and prevent friction and consequent skin breakdown and infection. They are made of cotton or wool and come in three weights: single ply, three ply, and five ply.

▶ NURSING DIAGNOSIS: *Impaired Physical Mobility*

Related To alterations in balance and loss of the lower extremity.

Defining Characteristics
Impaired ability to
- move self in bed
- transfer out of bed
- ambulate safely

Patient Outcomes
The patient will
- move self in bed to lateral, prone, and supine positions.
- transfer out of bed to chair or to walk.
- ambulate with assistance and/or assistive device.

Nursing Interventions	Rationales
Refer to prosthetist for application and care of prosthesis.	There are many types of prostheses available. The prosthetist is responsible for the fitting of the prosthesis and is knowledgeable about its application and care.
Refer to the physical therapist for preambulation exercises and gait training.	The physical therapist is an important member of the interdisciplinary team caring for patients with amputations.

Nursing Interventions

Teach patient to rewrap residual limb to promote shrinking and shaping:
1. Use a 4-in. elastic bandage and demonstrate a figure-eight wrapping technique, exerting the greatest amount of pressure over the end of the limb.
2. Keep the knee straight and wrap until the bandage is 3 or 4 in. above the knee.
3. Secure the bandage on the front of the thigh.
4. Reapply the bandage q4h during the day and anytime it is loose.

NOTE: A shrinker made of elasticized fabric may be used in place of the elastic bandage. This is applied like a stocking and goes 3–4 in. above the knee. The top may be folded (never rolled) down over the upper edge. The seam should stay in a straight line over the end of the limb. Reapply q4h during the day.

5. Either the bandage or shrinker is worn constantly except during bathing, after bathing when the residual limb is air drying, and when the prosthesis is worn. This procedure is continued until the limb retains its shape. This usually takes about 6 months.

Rationales

A prosthesis will not fit correctly if the residual limb is not properly shaped. If the patient elects to forego a prosthesis, an improperly shaped limb may become contracted and impair positioning and increase the risk for skin breakdown.

Instruct patient to position residual limb correctly [below-the-knee amputation (BKA)]:
1. Maintain knee in extension and do not prop knee with pillows or other devices.
2. Maintain hips in extension and adduction.

Incorrect positioning hastens the formation of flexion and abduction contractures.

Instruct patient to lie prone for 30 min a day.

Prone position facilitates extension of the hip and knee.

Nursing Interventions	**Rationales**

Instruct patient for chair-sitting:
1. below-the-knee amputation
  • without prosthesis: support residual limb on another chair or footstool of the same height; advise to sit upright, with weight equally distributed on both hips; tell to sit for not more than 2 h at a time
  • with prosthesis: sit with prosthetic foot forward with heel on floor and knee only partially flexed
2. above-the-knee amputation (AKA)
  • follow instructions for below the knee for bed positioning
  • for sitting without prosthesis: chair or footstool not necessary; do not prop limb on pillow
  • for sitting with prosthesis: keep legs in adduction and keep prosthetic foot flat on floor
	These interventions maintain body alignment with and without prosthesis.

Teach exercises (there are numerous other beneficial exercises; consult with physical therapist). Breathe normally while exercising and do exercises with residual limb and then with other leg:
 	
1. gluteal sets
  • lie on back and tighten buttocks; hold for a count of 5, relax, and repeat
  • place towel or pillow between thighs, while lying on back; with legs flat, squeeze towel or pillow, hold for a count of 5 and repeat
	These exercises strengthen and condition the residual limb.

Nursing Interventions	**Rationales**
2. sitting push-ups • while sitting up, do flexion of elbows and shoulders while holding a book or weight in each hand • sit up straight and raise arms straight out at sides at shoulder height with elbows straight; make small circles with both arms, going forward and then backward	These exercises strengthen the torso and upper extremities.
Instruct patient to move self in bed (side rails must be raised and bed flat): 1. moving to head of bed in supine position • remove pillow and place against head of bed • grasp side rails at shoulder level with hands; bend knee of intact leg and press foot into bed • lift buttocks and move body toward head of bed. **NOTE:** A trapeze may be used for this procedure. However, the consistent use of a trapeze for all bed activities may be detrimental because it does not promote conditioning of the triceps muscles. Strong triceps are needed for transfer and standing activities. 2. moving to left lateral position from supine position • move to right side of bed by grasping side rail at shoulder level on right side • bend knees and lift hips off bed and to right side; move leg and residual limb to the same side and, grasping side rail, pull shoulders to that side	Independent bed movement is the first step in progressive mobilization. It increases strength, endurance, and general body conditioning.

Nursing Interventions	Rationales

• if right leg is intact, cross this leg over residual limb
• reach across chest and grasp left side rail with right hand, pulling onto the side
3. moving to prone position from left lateral position
  • continue rolling when moving onto left side until prone position is reached
  • adjust position
4. moving to left lateral position from prone position
  • grasp side rail at shoulder height with right arm and roll onto side
  • reverse steps for moving to right lateral position	

Assist to transfer without prosthesis (use a one- or two-person assist depending on size and abilities of patient): 1. Prepare to transfer to side of strength. 2. Teach patient to turn over on side, flex knee on intact leg and to use arms to come to a sitting position. Leg(s) will automatically drop over side of bed as upper body comes to sitting position. 3. Assist, if necessary, by placing one arm over and around patient's knee(s) and the other arm around, under, and across patient's shoulders. 4. Apply transfer belt after patient comes to sitting position. 5. Place hands with underhand grasp in transfer belt and, on the count of 3, have patient move off edge of bed and come to standing position by side of bed.	Transferring out of bed provides the benefits of weight bearing on the unaffected leg. The active movement helps prevent complications associated with inactivity. Endurance and strength are increased.

Nursing Interventions

6. Maintain grasp on transfer belt. Instruct patient to pivot around until chair seat touches back of legs. Have patient reach for wheelchair arms with both hands and then gently lower into seat.

NOTE: The same procedure can be used with a prosthesis in place until the patient can independently transfer. A sliding board transfer can be taught to patients who are double amputees and who will not be wearing prostheses.

NOTE: Consult with physical therapist for ambulation. Instruct the patient in ambulating with a walker after the prosthesis is attached.

Apply a transfer belt and walk on the patient's affected side with one hand in the belt in underhand grasp until patient can safely maneuver alone.

1. Measure walker for proper size for patient.
2. Check rubber tips and screws for safety.
3. Tell patient to use a foot-over-foot, heel-strike gait.
4. Instruct patient to move walker ahead and then step into the walker with the prosthesis.
5. Follow with leg. Repeat the procedure.

Instruct patient to walk with cane:
1. Measure cane for proper fit and check cane for safety.
2. Start with cane in hand on *unaffected* side.
3. Move cane forward.
4. Move prosthesis forward.
5. Move unaffected leg forward. Repeat procedure.

Rationales

Prosthetic ambulation is preceded by building tolerance to weight bearing. The patient is not taught to walk until he or she can bear the amount of weight determined by the physician. Walking begins with parallel bars or a walker. Ambulating further increases strength and endurance. It increases the patient's endurance and self-esteem.

A cane is less cumbersome than a walker and further increases independence and patient abilities.

Nursing Interventions	Rationales

Advise patient to avoid situations that increase the risk of falling:
1. Provide with instructions for falling:
  • If prosthesis is not in place, walk on knees or scoot on buttocks to the closest sturdy object for support before attempting to stand.
  • With prosthesis attached, get up on hands and knees and then place unaffected foot flat on the floor. Push upward with hand and foot while bringing prosthesis forward.
  • Instruct patient to inspect both the prosthetic and unaffected leg after falling.
	The patient is not used to being limbless and may forget the limitations. The loss of a leg affects balance and coordination and it takes time to learn to compensate.

Clinical Clip

There should be no pain if there is a proper fit between the socket and residual limb. A competent prosthetist will fit the socket to the limb, not make a socket that the limb must endure.

▶ **NURSING DIAGNOSIS:** *Body Image Disturbance*

Related To loss of body part.

Defining Characteristics
• Avoids looking at or touching residual limb
• Change in ability to estimate spatial relationship of body to environment
• Feelings of helplessness, hopelessness, or powerlessness
• Fear of rejection by others
• Change in social involvement

Patient Outcomes
The patient will
• verbalize feelings about the amputation and self.
• participate in the care of the residual limb to the extent that he or she is able.

- express acceptance of changed body.
- seek information to regain independence.

Nursing Interventions	Rationales
Allow and assist patient to work through grief to facilitate acceptance of changed body.	Amputation of a body part drastically affects one's body image. Grieving for the lost part is a natural response and must be worked through to successful resolution.
Assign consistent caregivers. Actively listen to comments and encourage verbalization of feelings. Clarify areas of misunderstanding.	This will establish a therapeutic nurse-patient relationship.
Include the patient and significant other(s) in care planning.	Participation provides the patient with opportunity to make decisions, thereby increasing feelings of control. Including significant others facilitates interaction and mutual support.
Assist and encourage patient as necessary in activities of daily living, so that a well-groomed, attractive personal appearance is maintained.	Outward appearance can affect inner feelings about oneself.

DISCHARGE PLANNING/CONTINUITY OF CARE

The elderly patient with lower limb amputation may need further rehabilitation after leaving the acute-care setting. This may require transfer to a rehabilitation center or skilled nursing care facility: Inform the receiving facility of

- patient's mental and physical abilities.
- availability of patient's support system.
- progress concerning physical therapy.
- management of phantom sensations.

If patient is returning home,

- arrange for home health nurse to evaluate healing of residual limb.
- evaluate patient's/caregiver's ability to perform daily care of residual limb.
- evaluate patient's/caregiver's ability to identify signs and symptoms of complications.
- arrange for home or outpatient physical therapy services.
- complete home safety assessment (see Appendix B, page 343).

BIBLIOGRAPHY

Agency for Health Care Policy and Research. (1992). *Acute pain management: Operative or medical procedures and trauma.* Rockville, MD: U.S. Department of Health and Human Services.

Alexander, T. T. (1990). Procedures to maintain mobility. In C. E. Carlson, W. P. Griggs, & R. B. King (Eds.), *Rehabilitation nursing procedures manual.* Rockville, MD: Aspen.

DiDomenico, R. L., & Ziegler, W. Z. (1989). *Rehabilitation techniques for geriatric aides.* Rockville, MD: Aspen.

McCaffery, M., & Beebe, A. (1989). *Pain clinical manual for nursing practice.* St. Louis, MO: Mosby.

Marianjoy Rehabilitation Center. (1989). Training can ease phantom pain. *PhysiCare, September/October,* 4.

Nunnelee, J. D., Kurgan, A., & Auer, A. I. (1993). Distal bypasses in patients over age 75. *Geriatric Nursing, 14*(5), 252–254.

Swager, J. (1991). Musculoskeletal care. In M. Shaw (Ed.), *Illustrated manual of nursing practice.* Springhouse, PA: Springhouse Corporation.

Swearingen, P. L. (1992). *Pocket guide to medical-surgical nursing.* St. Louis, MO: Mosby Year-Book.

$\mathcal{H}$IP ARTHROPLASTY (PROSTHESIS)

Hip arthroplasty replaces both joint components. The degenerated femoral head is removed and a prosthetic head and intermedullary stem are inserted. A plastic or metal cup replaces the acetabulum. The components are cemented in place. The surgery relieves pain, restores motion, and enables the patient to resume activities.

ETIOLOGIES
- Degenerative arthritis of the hip
- Rheumatoid arthritis of the hip
- Femoral neck fracture

CLINICAL MANIFESTATIONS (PREOPERATIVELY)
- Severe, unrelenting pain not relieved by nonsteroidal anti-inflammatory drugs (NSAIDs)
- Loss of motion and functional deficits
- Adduction and external rotation of hip with shortening of the limb if fracture present

CLINICAL/DIAGNOSTIC FINDINGS (PREOPERATIVELY)
X-ray of hip showing degeneration or fracture

▶ NURSING DIAGNOSIS: *Impaired Physical Mobility*

Related To recent surgery and physician's orders for partial weight bearing and prior deconditioning.

Defining Characteristics
- Discomfort from surgery
- Inability to bear full weight

Patient Outcomes

The patient will participate in progressive mobility procedures and avoid dislocation of prosthesis.

Nursing Interventions	Rationales
Monitor operative site for the following: • swelling • redness or discoloration • severe pain • unusual positioning of affected extremity	These signs indicate dislocation of the prosthesis.
Implement 2-h positioning schedule: 1. Maintain hip abduction and avoid hip adduction. 2. Avoid internal and external hip rotation. Maintain hip in neutral position. Advise patient not to turn hip or knee inward or outward. 3. Turn to back and unaffected side only. Keep affected hip straight, with pillows to support affected limb when client is lying on side.	Frequent and correct repositioning prevents skin breakdown, contractures, and displacement of prosthesis.
Arrange bed so patient can get out of bed on unoperated side. Teach to roll onto side, use arms to support self, and gently swing both legs off the bed together. Place the bed high enough so the patient does not place stress on hip when rising from the side of the bed. Consult with physical therapist regarding weight bearing and use of assistive devices. Teach appropriate transfer techniques.	Avoid pressure on operated side. The amount of weight bearing and training for ambulation varies with the surgeon. Most patients use a walker and then progress to a cane. The nurse needs to know which gait the patient is to use with the device so that teaching can be reinforced and unsafe practices avoided. Some patients with rheumatoid arthritis find platform crutches less stressful to the joints of the arms than using a walker.
Maintain alignment of hip while patient is in chair, as indicated in intervention. Instruct patient to not cross the legs at any time and to avoid more than 90° hip flexion. Advise to sit in a chair with arms.	More than 90° flexion increases the risk of displacement of the prosthesis.

Nursing Interventions	Rationales
To come to a standing position from the chair, move to the edge of the chair, and place the unaffected leg back and affected leg forward. Use hands to push off the arms of the chair. Use raised toilet seat for bowel and bladder elimination.	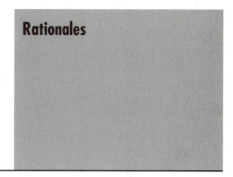

 NURSING DIAGNOSIS: *High Risk for Disuse Syndrome*

Risk Factors
- Reluctance to engage in physical activity due to fear of falling and reinjury
- Other health problems limiting mobility previous to surgery, such as arthritis and cardiac or pulmonary problems

Patient Outcomes
The patient will
- participate in activities of daily living (ADL).
- participate in diversional activities.
- be free of complications resulting from immobility.

Nursing Interventions	Rationales
Assess risk factors for complications that result from immobility: pressure ulcers, contractures, pneumonia, constipation, and incontinence.	Complications can be prevented by implementing preventive programs.
Encourage to do ADL as independently as possible. Arrange environment to facilitate independence: 1. Provide long-handled sponge for bathing. 2. Advise wearing shoes that can be put on without bending over. 3. Provide a dressing stick and sock/stocking assistive device. 4. Provide a reacher to obtain items that would otherwise	Adaptive devices allow patient to safely complete ADL with more independence. Use of these items avoids the need for bending. Increased independence provides motivation and boosts self-esteem.

Nursing Interventions	Rationales
require bending or stretching to obtain. 5. Provide with remote control for television.	
Encourage participation in activities of the patient's choice.	Cognitive and psychosocial activity is necessary for well-being and increases zest for living.

▶ NURSING DIAGNOSIS: *High Risk for Trauma (Fractures)*

Risk Factors
- Osteoporosis
- Risk factors for falling (see Osteoporosis, page 60)
- Impaired mobility

Patient Outcomes
The patient will
- utilize safe mobility techniques.
- reduce risk factors for falling.
- avoid injuries.

Nursing Interventions	Rationales
Assess mobility techniques frequently.	Mobility can be increased as abilities indicate.
Complete home safety assessment if patient is at home (see Home Safety Assessment, Appendix B).	The environment can be adapted to the safety needs of the patient, thus reducing the risk of falling.
See Osteoporosis, page 60, for additional interventions.	

▶ NURSING DIAGNOSIS: *Altered Thought Processes*

Related To
- Blood loss
- Aftereffects of anesthesia
- Sleep deprivation
- Sensory deprivation

- Drug side-effects
- Sudden dislocation of patient from home/nursing home to hospital, if surgery resulted from a fracture

Defining Characteristics

- Mental status changes
- Functional decline
- Disorientation
- Confusion

Patient Outcomes

The patient will remain calm and avoid experiencing agitation and anxiety associated with altered thought processes.

Nursing Interventions	Rationales
Assess current mental status to determine if disorientation is reversible or irreversible (see Mini Mental Status Examination, Appendix D, page 349).	If altered thought processes are reversible, interventions can be implemented to reduce the disorientation and confusion.
Evaluate laboratory data.	Electrolyte imbalance, inadequate nutritional status, vitamin and mineral deficiencies, metabolic disorders, and dehydration can all cause signs of dementia.
Monitor drug regime and drug history.	The elderly are at risk for drug interactions and side effects that cause signs of dementia.
Consult with family to determine previous mental status.	If patient has history of irreversible altered thought processes, the condition cannot be changed. Interventions are directed to avoiding agitation. (See Alzheimer's Disease, page 204.)
Implement measures to avoid complications: 1. Remove indwelling catheter if present. Implement bladder management program if necessary. 2. Reposition frequently as directed above. 3. Provide for adequate fluid intake. 4. Improve nutritional status if necessary.	Improving/maintaining healthy physical condition can minimize disorientation and confusion.

Nursing Interventions	Rationales
5. Instruct to cough and deep breathe.	
Assist patient to leave room at regular intervals throughout the day.	Sensory deprivation can result from remaining in the room 24 h a day. Sensory deprivation increases risk for disorientation.
Avoid the use of physical and chemical restraints.	There are physical and psychological consequences to the use of restraints that further increase disorientation.

DISCHARGE PLANNING/CONTINUITY OF CARE
- Provide instructions for preparation of home environment to prevent falls (see Home Safety Assessment, Appendix B, page 343).
- Advise to install raised toilet seat.
- Arrange for ongoing physical therapy if needed.
- Arrange for other services as needed for individual situation.

BIBLIOGRAPHY

Graham, C. (1993). Smart planning for joint replacement surgery. *Arthritis Today, 7*(4), 46–50.

O'Brien, L. A., Grisso, J. A., Maislin, G., Chiu, G. Y., & Evans, L. (1993). Confusion and hip fracture. *Journal of Gerontological Nursing, 19*(2), 25–31.

Stevens, K. A. (1990). Hip Precautions. In C. E. Carlson, W. P. Griggs, & R. B. King (Eds.) *Rehabilitation Nursing Procedures Manual.* (pp. 272–273). Rockville, MD: Aspen Publishers, Inc.

OSTEOPOROSIS

During the first 30 years of life, there is a constant process of bone formation and resorption (remodeling). The loss of existing bone (resorption) is coupled with the formation of new bone. In the third or fourth decade, the process becomes uncoupled. During the aging process some loss of bone is expected. When the loss becomes severe, it is called osteoporosis. The reduction in bone mass presents a high risk of nontraumatic fractures.

ETIOLOGIES
The etiology of osteoporosis is unclear. It is associated with
- estrogen deficiency associated with menopause.
- reduced calcium intake.

There are several known risk factors:
- female sex
- white race
- family history
- small stature
- low levels of weight-bearing activity
- heavy cigarette smoking
- heavy alcohol use
- chronic conditions affecting the gastrointestinal, pulmonary, renal, hepatic, and endocrine systems
- chronic administration of glucocorticoids

CLINICAL MANIFESTATIONS
There are no obvious clinical manifestations until the disease is advanced:
- loss of tooth support resulting from mandibular alveolar bone loss
- significant loss of height
- kyphosis (dowager's hump)
- noted on x-ray when spontaneous fracture occurs

CLINICAL/DIAGNOSTIC FINDINGS

These diagnostic procedures reveal calcium loss from the bones if osteoporosis is present:

- computerized tomography (CT) scan
- dual-photon absorptiometer
- single-photon absorptiometer

▶ NURSING DIAGNOSIS: *High Risk for Trauma (Fractures)*

Risk Factors

- Internal (related to osteoporosis, aging changes, and other health problems)
  - brittleness and fragility of bones
  - impaired balance and coordination
  - sensory changes; vision and hearing
  - decreased blood supply to lower extremities
  - decreased strength and endurance
  - degenerative changes of joints
  - increased reaction time
  - orthostatic hypotension
  - medications affecting sensorium
- External: unsafe conditions of
  - floors/walking surfaces
  - lighting
  - furniture arrangements
  - clothing

Patient Outcomes

The patient will

- reduce risk factors that can be controlled.
- utilize safe behaviors to diminish the risk of falling.

Nursing Interventions	Rationales
Assess patient to determine the presence of risk factors for fractures.	Interventions can be planned to compensate for or remove the risk factors.
Instruct to 1. avoid sudden, quick movements. 2. sit on the edge of the bed for a few moments before arising. 3. put on glasses and insert hearing aid before getting out of bed.	These measures avoid orthostatic hypotension, which is a major cause of falls in the elderly. Wearing prescribed glasses and hearing aid improves balance and coordination.

Nursing Interventions	Rationales
Evaluate presence of risk factors for osteoporosis.	By identifying presence of risk factors, changes in life-style may be implemented that will decrease the risk factors for osteoporosis.

Work with patient to establish interventions/changes to reduce risk factors:
1. cessation of smoking
2. increasing calcium intake and calorie level if necessary to maintain body weight within the norm for age and body structure
3. avoiding alcohol
4. establishing exercise program:
  • a daily 30-min walk will increase strength and endurance and increase blood supply to lower extremities
  • daily stretching exercises will maintain joint flexibility
5. correcting underlying physiological problems
6. establishing bladder management program if patient is incontinent
	Reducing risk factors reduces the risk of fractures.

Suggest consultation with physician regarding administration of estrogen replacement therapy (ERT).	Some investigators recommend ERT beginning at menopause and continuing for 15 years. There is no definitive evidence that beginning ERT after age 70 is beneficial. The risk of breast cancer associated with ERT remains controversial.

External (patient):
1. Instruct patient to
  • use correct transfer techniques when moving from chair to another surface.
  • wear well-fitting, nonskid shoes and avoid shoelaces if possible. Advise shufflers to wear nonslip shoes that glide safely on floor.
	Falls in the elderly are frequently a result of faulty transfer techniques or the wrong clothing. In the institutional setting, dependent patients may attempt to get up to meet a physical need (i.e., going to the bathroom).

Nursing Interventions	Rationales

• check pants/slacks for length and shorten if necessary.
• avoid walking in robes.
• remove throw rugs.
• avoid climbing on chairs to reach items.
• place nightlight in bathroom and bedroom.
2. Additional interventions in hospital/long-term care facility include:
  • attending to unmet physiological needs promptly.
  • alerting staff if patient has taken a laxative or diuretic.
  • maintaining bed in lowest position.
  • keeping call bell within reach.
  • placing nightlight in room.	

External (environmental) (see Home Safety Assessment, Appendix B, page 343).	A safe environment reduces the risk for falling.
Implement a restraint reduction program in hospital/long-term care facility.	Restraints should never be used to prevent a patient from walking. The use of restraints increases incidents and injuries and diminishes self-esteem.

▶ NURSING DIAGNOSIS: *Altered Nutrition—Less Than Body Requirements (Calcium)*

Related To
• Lack of information
• Poor dietary habits

Defining Characteristics
• Nutritional history indicating insufficient intake of calcium
• Medical diagnosis of osteoporosis

Patient Outcomes
The patient will
• verbalize knowledge of calcium need and foods high in calcium.
• increase calcium intake by eating foods high in calcium.

Nursing Interventions	Rationales
Assess food likes and dislikes.	It is pointless to suggest foods high in calcium if the patient will not eat them.
Advise choosing adequate amounts of these foods daily: 1. dark, green leafy vegetables 2. low-fat dairy products: skim milk, yogurt, low-fat cheese 3. salmon 4. tofu 5. almonds	A daily minimum of 800 mg of calcium is recommended for all adults. The recommended daily intake of calcium for all post-menopausal women and for older men is 1,000–1,500 mg. Eating a variety of high-calcium foods will ensure adequate calcium intake.
Advise patient to avoid eating calcium-rich foods and high-fiber foods together.	Fiber prevents calcium absorption.
Advise patient to consume adequate amounts of protein and vitamin D. Eating a well-balanced diet meeting daily recommendations should provide adequate amounts.	Protein is needed for strong bones; excessively high levels can aggravate bone loss. Vitamin D is needed to facilitate calcium absorption, but megadoses are toxic.
Advise to take calcium supplements if prescribed. (Some researchers believe that in postmenopausal women calcium is only effective if taken in conjunction with ERT.)	Calcium supplements should only be taken when adequate amounts of dietary calcium cannot be consumed.
Calcium carbonate is the best supplement. Calcium should be taken with meals with 10–20 ounces of water with each calcium tablet.	Calcium carbonate has the largest concentration of calcium. Bone meal and dolomite are potential sources of lead poisoning and should not be used. Absorption is better in persons over 60 years if calcium is taken with meals.

DISCHARGE PLANNING/CONTINUITY OF CARE
- Arrange for meals-on-wheels if patient is unable to purchase and prepare nutritionally balanced meals.
- Suggest renting a telephone service that is programmed to signal for help if the patient falls.
- Assess for environmental safety (see Appendix B, page 343).

Clinical Clip

Nearly 200,000 women suffer hip fractures every year as a result of osteoporosis. Twenty percent of these women will die of complications within the first year. Twenty-five percent of women over 60 years have fractured vertebra, limiting activities and leading to kyphosis.

BIBLIOGRAPHY

Ali, N. S., & Bennett, S. J. (1992). Postmenopausal women: Factors in osteoporosis preventive behaviors. *Journal of Gerontological Nursing, 18*(12), 23–32.

Dairy Council. (1991, April). *Nutrition newsbreak*. Paper presented at International Consensus Conference on Osteoporosis.

McMahon, M. A., Peterson, C., & Schilke, J. (1992). Osteoporosis: Identifying high-risk persons. *Journal of Gerontological Nursing, 18*(10), 19–26.

Sardana, R. (1992). Nutritional management of osteoporosis. *Geriatric Nursing, 13*(6), 315–319.

Special Committee on Aging, United States Senate. (1990). *Untie the elderly: Quality care without restraints*. Serial No. 101-H. Washington, DC: U.S. Government Printing Office.

$\mathscr{R}$HEUMATOID ARTHRITIS

$\mathbf{R}$heumatoid arthritis (RA) is an inflammatory, systemic disease of unknown cause often characterized by remissions and exacerbations. Varying degrees of disability are associated with RA depending on the progression and severity of the disease. A small number of people develop joint deformities resulting from swelling and inflammation of the synovial membrane. Because the disease is systemic, other organs and body systems can be affected.

ETIOLOGIES
The cause is unknown, but it is thought to develop and perpetuate as a result of an autoimmune disorder.

CLINICAL MANIFESTATIONS
- Joint involvement
  - soreness, aching, warmth over joints
  - stiffness upon arising for 30 min to 2 h and after long periods of inactivity
  - joints of hands and feet affected first
  - symmetrical joint involvement
  - painless, movable rheumatoid nodules often found over pressure points
- Anorexia
- Slight loss of weight
- Fatigue
- Deficits, instrumental activities of daily living (IADL)

CLINICAL/DIAGNOSTIC FINDINGS
- Erythrocyte sedimentation rate elevated in 80–90% of patients
- Rheumatoid factor is positive in 75–80% of patients with a titer >1:160 or higher
- Red blood cell (RBC) count <4.7 × 10^6/mm^3 in men, <4.2 × 10^6/mm^3 in women
- Hemoglobin (Hgb) <14 g/dL in men, <12 g/dL in women
- Hematocrit (Hct) <42% in men, <37% in women

- Cryoglobulin test: globulin levels between 1 and 5 mm associated with RA
- Leukocyte count elevated >10,000 mm^3 during inflammatory periods
- Deteriorating joint changes over time shown on x-ray

▶ NURSING DIAGNOSIS: *Chronic Pain*

Related To inflammation of synovial membrane.

Defining Characteristics
- Verbal expression of pain
- Guarding behavior of affected joint
- Inability to perform activities of daily living (ADL)
- Withdrawal from social and physical activities
- Changes in sleep pattern

Patient Outcomes
The patient will
- experience relief of pain, as evidenced by
  - verbal expression.
  - ability to perform ADL.
  - resuming previous social and physical activities.
  - resuming previous sleep pattern.
- verbalize knowledge of prescribed medications and nonpharmacologic pain-relieving strategies.

Nursing Interventions	Rationales
Administer nonsteroidal anti-inflammatory drugs (NSAIDs) as prescribed: 1. Give medication four times daily. 2. Administer with food or antacids. 3. Check renal and hepatic function periodically. 4. Instruct patient to report blood in stools or black, tarry stools, visual disturbances, edema, or weight gain.	Pain relief is more successful if medication is administered routinely rather than as needed. The NSAIDs are absorbed more efficiently and are less irritating to the stomach when given with food or antacids. Side effects of NSAIDs may affect the kidneys, liver, or gastrointestinal or central nervous systems.

Nursing Interventions	Rationales
Teach patient to rate pain and evaluate effectiveness of medication using a scale of 0 (no pain) to 10 (severe pain).	Patient is given a sense of control. Pain relief is more effectively evaluated by the patient.
Plan for a 30-min rest period after medication is given before proceeding with physical activity.	A routine that alternates periods of rest with periods of activity prevents stiffness associated with rest and pain associated with lengthy physical activity.
Teach the use of progressive relaxation techniques using a pre-recorded tape of instructions in a quiet, private area.	Muscle relaxation interrupts the cycle of pain, anxiety, and muscle tension, which perpetuate each other. Relaxation enhances the effect of the pain medication.
Administer moist heat and/or cold treatments twice a day.	Both modalities are used for temporary relief of joint pain. Cold compresses are more effective for acute pain resulting from hot, painful joints. Heat is used for subacute or chronic joint problems. Moist heat penetrates joints deeper. Either modality works better when administered intermittently for short periods rather than for long periods only once a day.

▶ **NURSING DIAGNOSIS:** *High Risk for Disuse Syndrome*

Risk Factors
- Joint pain and stiffness
- Belief that constant rest is beneficial to pain
- Decreasing functional abilities

Patient Outcomes
The patient will
- comply with rest/activity routine.
- maintain previous/present functional abilities.

Nursing Interventions	Rationales
Change position in bed at least q2h. Keep bed flat to avoid positions of flexion. Assist to lie in prone position for 15 min four times a day if possible (allow feet to hang over end of mattress). Note chair-sitting position and provide positioning devices to maintain body alignment.	Stiffness, pain, and contractures can be prevented by maintaining joints in extension. Lying in prone position enables all joints to be in extension. Plantar flexion is avoided when feet hang over end of mattress.
Instruct/assist in exercise techniques: 1. active or active-assistive range-of-motion (ROM) exercises twice a day, starting with slow, gentle stretch and moving each joint through its full range 2. isometric exercises 3. endurance exercises: ambulation, alternating periods of brisk walking with periods of leisurely pacing, gradually increasing the distance	Range-of-motion exercises maintain functional use of the extremities and prevent pain, stiffness, and contractures. Isometric exercises strengthen and maintain joint stability. Endurance exercises promote cardiovascular fitness, thus avoiding general deterioration. NOTE: Adaptations must be made to the exercise interventions during an acute phase of the disease. Exercise may be limited to passive ROM.
Consult with physical therapist, occupational therapist, or physician regarding need for orthosis (splint) of hand(s).	An orthosis may prevent or delay deformities of the fingers by maintaining the joints in functional position.

▶ NURSING DIAGNOSIS: *Fatigue*

Related To
- Increased energy requirements to perform ADL
- Increased metabolic demands during inflammatory periods
- Chronic pain

Defining Characteristics
- Verbalization of constant lack of energy
- Inability to maintain usual activity level

Patient Outcomes
The patient will
- verbalize an increased energy level.
- perform usual activities.

Nursing Interventions	Rationales
Establish a structured routine that alternates exercise with rest: 1. toileting upon awakening, medications with milk 2. ROM exercises with gentle stretching 3. rest 4. morning care 5. rest 6. breakfast 7. heat treatments 8. rest and relaxation techniques 9. ambulation 10. rest 11. activity of choice 12. lunch and medication 13. rest 14. exercise: ROM, gentle stretching, isometrics 15. rest 16. dinner and medication 17. rest 18. ambulation 19. rest 20. activity of choice 21. medication with light snack, rest 22. bedtime care	Prevent pain from overuse of joints and prevent stiffness that results from prolonged periods of inactivity.
Teach modifying techniques and provide adaptive aids to use when completing ADL: 1. Utilize adaptive handles for combs, brushes, pencils, and eating utensils. 2. Use a rubber gripper for turning on faucets. 3. Use electrical appliances when possible: toothbrush, can opener.	The handles provide an easier grip if the hand and fingers cannot be fully flexed and reduce stress on the joints.
Use long-handled items such as a reacher, shoehorn, zipper pull, stocking aid, button aid, and dressing stick.	The need to reach is avoided.

Nursing Interventions	Rationales
Provide a shower seat or tub chair for bathing.	Energy expenditure is less.
Perform activities while seated if possible.	

▶ NURSING DIAGNOSIS: *Diversional Activity Deficit*

Related To inability to participate in former hobbies and pastimes.

Defining Characteristics
Expressions of dissatisfaction with lack of hobbies and pastimes.

Patient Outcomes
The patient will participate in activities within physical capabilities and personal choice.

Nursing Interventions	Rationales
Discuss previous hobbies and pastimes.	Adaptations may be made to allow participation, for example, using a card holder and automatic shuffler for card playing.
Discuss activities that require only passive participation such as listening to music.	These provide enjoyment without expenditure of energy.
Offer new activities that are physically realistic.	Exploring new ideas may open up a new realm of interest that would not otherwise be tapped.

DISCHARGE PLANNING/CONTINUITY OF CARE
- Provide suggestions for organizing the home for efficiency and to minimize fatigue.
- Suggest participation in a self-help program sponsored by the Arthritis Foundation.
- Offer to enlist the services of a homemaker program to provide assistance with household tasks so that energy can be used for activities of the patient's choice.

Clinical Clip

- Researchers at the Mayo Clinic have found a genetic marker for RA. People who inherit this sequence from both parents are more likely to develop RA.

- Patient education can improve life for persons with RA. Evidence from 76 studies shows increases in patient knowledge, increases in positive behaviors, and improved health outcomes after patient education.

Table 8.1 • Comparison of Rheumatoid Arthritis and Osteoarthritis (OA)

	RA	OA
Description	Autoimmune reaction Joint inflammation Systemic disease	Degeneration of cartilage and other joint tissues No inflammation Localized
Cause	Most people with RA have genetic marker Family history	Wear and tear Joint injury
Incidence	3% of adult population 7 million in U.S. Three-fourths are women Average age of onset, 35 years	17 million people Twice as many women as men Onset, over age 40
Clinical manifestations	Swelling, heat, redness Limitation of function Bilateral, symmetrical Starts in hands, feet, then larger joints Rheumatoid nodules on scalp, ear, ulna, olecranon, heels Sjögren's syndrome may be present Pain worse in a.m. Exacerbations/remissions or only few attacks or slowly progressive Ankylosis occurs in severe cases	No heat or redness No limitation of function unless degeneration is severe No constant symptoms of any specific joint Heberden's nodes, Bouchard's nodes Morning stiffness is brief, alleviated with shower, exercise Pain alleviated with rest, but stiffness sets in with rest Pain affected by weather Ankylosis does not occur

Table 8.1 • *continued*

	RA	OA
Clinical/diagnostic findings	C reactive protein, positive Sedimentation rate increased Latex fixation and antinuclear antibodies are positive X-ray shows erosion of bone, tissue swelling	No definitive laboratory test History
Interventions	NSAIDs Aspirin Corticosteroids Gold treatment Penicillamine Cytotoxic drugs Heat/cold treatments Balance of rest/exercise Joint protection techniques	NSAIDs Aspirin Heat and cold treatments Exercise/rest Joint protection techniques

BIBLIOGRAPHY

Acute pain management. Operative or medical procedures and trauma. (1992). Agency for Health Care Policy and Research. U.S. Department of Health and Human Services. Rockville, MD.

Arthritis Foundation Illinois. (1993a). *News item.* Spring 1993, p. 5. Chicago.

Arthritis Foundation Illinois. (1993b). *Gene may predict severity in rheumatoid arthritis.* Fall 1993, p. 1. Chicago.

McCaffery, M., & Beebe, A. (1989). *Pain control manual for nursing practice.* St. Louis, MO: Mosby.

Mirabelli, L. (1990). Caring for patients with rheumatoid arthritis. *Nursing 90, 20*(9), 67, 68, 70, 72.

Cardiovascular Conditions

CHRONIC CONGESTIVE HEART FAILURE

Congestive heart failure (CHF) is one cause of decreased cardiac output and occurs when the heart is unable to pump sufficient blood to meet the metabolic needs of the body. Cardiac output is the heart rate multiplied by the stroke volume. Stroke volume is the quantity of blood ejected from the ventricles with each contraction and depends on preload, afterload, and contractility. Preload is the force that stretches the heart muscle during diastole. Afterload is the pressure the ventricles must overcome to open the aortic and pulmonic valves and pump blood out of the heart. Contractility is the intensity with which the heart muscle contracts. Congestive heart failure can be acute or chronic and either left sided or right sided or mixed.

ETIOLOGIES
- Hypertension
- Cardiomyopathy
- Valvular disease
- Ischemic heart disease
- Congenital heart defects
- Rheumatic heart disease
- Chronic obstructive pulmonary disease (COPD)

CLINICAL MANIFESTATIONS
- Left-sided failure (diastolic heart failure)
  - increased heart rate
  - exertional dyspnea, possibly paroxysmal nocturnal dyspnea, Cheyne-Stokes respirations, orthopnea
  - pale, cool skin
  - arrhythmias
  - fatigue
  - shortened attention span, restlessness, irritability

- Right-sided failure (systolic heart failure)
  - –increased heart rate
  - –edema
  - –distended, rigid neck veins
  - –hepatomegaly
  - –occasional ascites
  - –cyanosis
  - –arrhythmias
  - –dyspnea

CLINICAL/DIAGNOSTIC FINDINGS

- Echocardiogram (ECG): Left- and right-sided heart failure—valvular disorders, ventricular hypertrophy, decreased contractility
- Multigated blood pool imaging (MUGA): left ventricular abnormalities
- Exercise stress thallium or persantine thallium for patients who cannot exercise for thallium stress test: ischemia due to coronary artery disease
- Electrocardiogram (EKG): tachycardia and extra systoles
- Cardiac catheterization: coronary artery disease
- Chest x-ray: cardiomegaly, pleural effusion

▶ NURSING DIAGNOSIS: *Decreased Cardiac Output*

Related To ineffective pumping of the heart.

Defining Characteristics

- Variations in blood pressure readings
- Arrhythmias
- Fatigue
- Jugular vein distention
- Color changes in skin and mucous membranes
- Oliguria
- Dyspnea, orthopnea, restlessness
- Cold, clammy skin
- Rales
- Decreased peripheral pulses

Patient Outcomes

The patient will

- maintain stable blood pressure and pulse rate.
- exhibit increased physical endurance.
- experience decreased respiratory distress.

Nursing Interventions	Rationales
Administer digoxin as prescribed.	Digoxin strengthens the heart muscle and contractility by facilitating movement of calcium from extracellular to intracellular cytoplasm

Nursing Interventions	Rationales
	and inhibiting sodium-potassium activated adenosine triphosphatase (ADT). This action strengthens the heart muscle and contractility, thus increasing cardiac output.
Monitor serum digitalis levels. Therapeutic plasma level is 0.5–2.0 mg/mL. Monitor K$^+$ (potassium) levels.	Seventy percent of digoxin is excreted through the kidneys. The aged are at risk for digoxin toxicity because kidney function is significantly diminished. Therapeutic levels for digitalis are narrow. Advancing heart disease further decreases the margin. Elevated K$^+$ levels increase arrhythmias. Decreased K$^+$ levels enhance digoxin toxicity.
Take the apical pulse for 1 min routinely and before administration of digoxin. Notify physician of significant changes: 1. sudden increase or decrease in rate 2. pulse deficit (the difference between apical and peripheral pulses) 3. irregular beats 4. regularization of a previously irregular rhythm	Digitalis levels alone may not present an accurate picture. Persons sensitive to digitalis may present symptoms of toxicity when levels are below the therapeutic range. Clinical signs and symptoms must be considered with the digitalis levels for accurate assessment.

Monitor blood pressure and lung sounds. Notify physician and obtain 12-lead EKG for these changes. Teach patient to take pulse. Advise patient to report signs of digoxin toxicity:
1. anorexia
2. nausea and vomiting
3. diarrhea
4. visual disturbances
  • yellow-green halos around images
  • blurred or double vision
	Gastrointestinal and central nervous system (CNS) symptoms are usually the first signs of toxicity and may precede cardiac symptoms. Increased severity of CHF is an adverse reaction to digoxin and must be identified at onset for rapid resolution.

Nursing Interventions	Rationales
• light flashes 5. weakness 6. fatigue 7. mood alterations 8. changes in pulse rate and rhythm	
Monitor electrolyte levels.	Digitalis toxicity may be acceler-ated by hypokalemia and may be exacerbated by hypomagnesemia and hypercalcemia.
Monitor blood urea nitrogen (BUN) and creatinine levels.	Because elderly patients have diminished kidney function, digi-talis is not excreted as efficiently as in a younger person. The BUN lev-els alone do not always present an accurate picture of kidney function in the elderly. The significance of the BUN, creatinine levels, digitalis levels, and clinical manifestations are considered together.

▶ NURSING DIAGNOSIS: *Fluid Volume Excess*

Related To low cardiac output and blood backup behind one or both ventricles.

Defining Characteristics
• Edema
• Weight gain
• Shortness of breath
• Orthopnea
• Fluid intake greater than fluid output
• Pulmonary congestion
• Rales

Patient Outcomes
The patient will
• maintain a stable weight.
• have an absence of edema.
• experience less respiratory discomfort.
• maintain a balanced fluid intake and output.
• have an absence of rales and pulmonary congestion.

Nursing Interventions	Rationales
Administer furosemide as prescribed.	Furosemide increases water excretion by increasing sodium ion excretion.
Monitor blood pressure and heart rate during rapid diuresis. Monitor serum electrolytes, BUN, and CO_2 frequently.	Potency of medication can lead to water and electrolyte depletion. Elderly patients are at risk for excessive diuresis resulting in circulatory collapse, thrombosis, and embolus.
Monitor for hypokalemia. Monitor for and instruct patient to report the following: 1. muscle weakness and cramps 2. twitching 3. irregular heartbeat 4. hypoactive reflexes 5. paresthesia 6. confusion 7. nausea and vomiting 8. diarrhea Monitor K^+ levels. Instruct patient to eat potassium-rich foods: apricots, bananas, citrus fruits, dates, tomatoes.	Diuresis diminishes K^+ levels. Low K^+ levels predispose to digitalis toxicity.
Weigh daily in the morning after voiding and before breakfast and on the same scale. Report weight gain over 1 kg (2.2 lb) if food intake has not been increased. Limit fluid intake to 1,000–1,500 mL daily.	Weight is the most accurate assessment of daily fluid balance. For example, 2.2 kg is equivalent to 1 L of fluid retention. Limiting fluid intake decreases the risk of fluid overload.
Observe lower extremities, hips, and back for signs of edema.	Fluid retention may be evident in less obvious body tissues, causing pressure on nerves and resulting in pain.
Assist to identify high- and low-sodium foods. Explain why it is beneficial to avoid high dietary sodium intake. Caution against overuse of salt substitutes.	Increased sodium level causes fluid retention. Sodium intake can be lowered by avoiding high-sodium foods in the diet. Most salt substitutes contain potassium. Potassium is excreted through the kidneys

Nursing Interventions

Rationales

and elderly persons with diminished kidney function may retain large amounts of potassium, leading to hyperkalemia.

▶ **NURSING DIAGNOSIS:** *Activity Intolerance*

Related To alterations in oxygen delivery to body tissues due to decreased cardiac output and resulting in anginal pain.

Defining Characteristics
- Verbal report of fatigue, weakness, and anginal pain
- Abnormal heart rate or blood pressure response to activity
- Exertional dyspnea

Patient Outcomes
The patient will
- pace self to avoid fatigue, shortness of breath, and anginal pain.
- report any increase in fatigue, shortness of breath, chest pain, headache, or dizziness.
- be able to participate in chosen activities.

Nursing Interventions	Rationales
Assess pulse before and after getting out of bed. Monitor for signs or complaints of weakness, fatigue, shortness of breath, or chest pain. If chest pain is present, take blood pressure, auscultate lungs and heart, and note duration, intensity, and location of pain and presence of diuresis.	Adverse signs are indications of severity of heart disease. Activity level may need to be modified.
Place commode at bedside for use during night.	Use of a commode rather than a bedpan maintains independence, facilitates emptying of bladder, and reduces energy expenditures.
Advise that increased activity on a good day may result in additional fatigue the next day.	Careful planning may allow the patient to tolerate more activity.

Nursing Interventions	Rationales
Allow to proceed at own pace and to rest as soon as fatigue is experienced.	Self-regulation of activities can increase quality of life.
Plan nursing care to allow for periods of rest before and after activity/care.	Allowing the patient to become overfatigued due to nursing care diminishes the patient's ability to participate in activities of choice.
Encourage to maintain regular physical activity, such as walking, within the limits of endurance.	Regular exercise within the patient's limits prevents deconditioning associated with inactivity.
Advise to use wheelchair to allow fuller participation in activities of choice, for example, shopping in a mall.	The patient needs to know that favorite activities may be allowable with adaptations.
Administer nitrates as prescribed. There are four types: 1. erythritol tetranitrate 2. isosorbide dinitrate 3. pentaerythritol tetranitrate 4. glyceryl trinitrate (nitroglycerin) Nitroglycerin may be administered as follows: 5. sublingual 6. oral 7. buccal 8. transmucosal 9. sublingual sprays 10. transdermal discs or pads 11. ointment 12. intravenous Nitrates may be administered as prophylaxis for chronic pain or before stressful events to prevent/minimize pain, depending on the type that is prescribed. All forms may be used prophylactically. Sublingual tablets, lingual sprays, buccal tablets, and intravenous administration are the only forms appropriate for treatment of acute angina.	Nitrates are commonly prescribed for persons with ischemic heart disease to manage the pain of angina pectoris. Nitroglycerin decreases preload in left ventricle and afterload, thus reducing cardiac oxygen demand. Blood flow through collateral coronary vessels is increased. Acute anginal pain is relieved.

Nursing Interventions	Rationales
Monitor effectiveness of drug.	Tolerance to nitroglycerin develops with some forms of the medication. A nitrate-free interval is recommended with 1. immediate-release isosorbide dinitrate. 2. sustained-release isosorbide dinitrate. 3. buccal nitroglycerin. 4. sustained-release nitroglycerin. 5. nitroglycerin ointment and patches. 6. nitroglycerin infusions. NOTE: The nitrate-free interval can be at night for patients who do not have anginal pain at that time. If nocturnal chest pains occur, the nitrate-free period can be scheduled during the day or a beta-adrenergic blocker or calcium channel blocker could be considered.
Monitor for adverse reactions: headache, dizziness, orthostatic hypotension, tachycardia, flushing, and palpitations.	Nitroglycerin acts directly on vascular, smooth muscle. If patient is taking other medication that directly or indirectly acts on vascular smooth muscle, there may be an increased or decreased effect depending on the medication. Signs of tachycardia or hypotension may indicate a dosage that is too high.
Instruct patient to 1. take medication regularly as prescribed. 2. take/apply medication as specific form of medication indicates. 3. be able to name medications, actions, dosage, and side effects. 4. avoid alcoholic beverages.	The medication is most effective and pain is better controlled when patient is knowledgeable and is able to manage administration.

Nursing Interventions

5. avoid orthostatic hypotension: rise to sitting or to standing position slowly and to sit back down if dizziness is experienced.
6. report signs and symptoms of adverse reactions described above.
7. store medication as indicated by specific form of drug.
8. keep a record of when the pain occurs and how much medication is required to relieve pain.

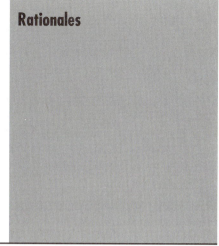

▶ **NURSING DIAGNOSIS:** *Altered Role Performance*

Related To inability to perform usual tasks due to activity intolerance.

Defining Characteristics
- Change in capacity to resume role
- Change in usual patterns of responsibility

Patient Outcomes
The patient will
- verbalize realistic self-expectations in consideration of limitations imposed by disease.
- discuss situation with family and make necessary adaptations.
- continue with activities that are within capabilities.

Nursing Interventions	Rationales
Assess patient's perceptions about current situation.	The patient may view self as totally helpless and generate a pattern of continuing physical and mental deterioration; or the patient may deny limitations and experience increasing levels of frustration related to activity intolerance.
Discuss with patient/family 1. the previous responsibilities of the patient.	Self-esteem is closely related to one's ability to fulfill role expectations. There may also be cultural

Nursing Interventions	Rationales
2. which responsibilities/activities are important to the patient. 3. whether or not these responsibilities/activities can safely be pursued. 4. adaptations that can be made in order to allow the patient to resume previous activities of choice.	factors related to the way in which the patient/family adapts to the situation. It is beneficial to the patient to meet self-expectations within the limits of the individual's abilities.
Provide the patient with opportunities to discuss concerns about sexuality.	Sexuality is a life-long need for both men and women and may or may not include sexual intercourse. The patient may be reluctant to ask questions, so it is important to facilitate open communication. If the patient is sexually active, counseling may be needed for both partners, in order to allow them to safely resume sexual activity. If necessary, encourage the patient/partner to consider alternatives to intercourse and to appreciate the rewards of intimacy.

DISCHARGE PLANNING/CONTINUITY OF CARE

- Assess the need for community resources:
  - home health nurse to periodically evaluate patient's condition and to draw blood for monitoring digitalis levels, electrolyte levels, BUN, and creatinine
  - home health aide to assist with activities of daily living
  - home-delivered meals
  - homemaker to assist with routine daily household chores
- Evaluate patient's/caregiver's knowledge regarding
  - administration of medications, their side effects, and signs and symptoms of toxicity.
  - ability to take pulse.
  - dietary management and fluid intake restrictions.
  - need for blood pressure monitoring.
  - energy conservation techniques.

Clinical Clip

Dynamic cardiomyoplasty is palliative surgery for patients with severe CHF due to irreversible cardiomyopathy. It does not replace a transplant but may be an alternative for persons who are not transplant candidates. Muscle from the back is used to restructure the myocardium and is then conditioned to augment ventricular contractions.

BIBLIOGRAPHY

Bushnell, F. K. L. (1992). Self-care teaching for congestive heart failure patients. *Journal of Gerontological Nursing, 18*(10), 27–32.

Cooke, D. M. (1992). Shielding your patient from digitalis toxicity. *Nursing 92, 22*(7), 44–47.

Hochrein, M., & Sohl, L. (1992). Heart smart: A guide to cardiac tests. *American Journal of Nursing, 92*(12), 22–25.

Letterer, R. A., Carew, B., Reid, M., & Woods, P. (1992). Learning to live with congestive heart failure. *Nursing 92, 22*(5), 34–41.

Wyatt, D. M. (1993). Dynamic cardiomyoplasty. *Nursing 93, 23*(7), 32u, 32y, 32z, 32bb.

Yakabowich, M. (1992). What you should know about administering nitrates. *Nursing 92, 22*(9), 52–55.

$\mathcal{H}$YPERTENSION

Hypertension is a major health problem in this country, and the incidence rises with age. Hypertension is a major risk factor for stroke, so alleviating this risk factor reduces the incidence of stroke. The National Institutes of Health recommends lifestyle modifications as the basis for hypertension control. If blood pressure remains at or above 140/90 mm Hg for 3–6 months despite these changes, then drug therapy needs to be implemented.

ETIOLOGIES
- Researchers have proposed various causes for hypertension:
  - high circulating insulin levels
  - insufficient opioids secreting during stressful situations
  - abnormality of the renal–body fluid control system
  - abnormality of the renin-angiotensin system
- There are several risk factors associated with hypertension:
  - obesity, especially abdominal obesity
  - smoking
  - lack of exercise
  - excessive alcohol consumption
  - diabetes mellitus

CLINICAL MANIFESTATIONS
Hypertension is a "silent" disease. Elevated blood pressure is usually noted upon routine physical examination.

CLINICAL/DIAGNOSTIC FINDINGS
Take blood pressure in both arms and use the arm with the higher reading for all succeeding measurements. Hypertension has recently been classified into four stages of the disease:

Stage 1	systolic 140–159 mm Hg	diastolic 90–99 mm Hg
Stage 2	systolic 160–179 mm Hg	diastolic 100–109 mm Hg
Stage 3	systolic 180–209 mm Hg	diastolic 110–119 mm Hg
Stage 4	systolic ≥ 210 mm Hg	diastolic ≥ 120 mm Hg

▶ **NURSING DIAGNOSIS:** *Altered Nutrition—More Than Body Requirements*

Related To excessive food intake and insufficient exercise.

Defining Characteristics
- Weight 10–20% over ideal for height and frame
- Triceps skin fold (TSF) >15 mm in men, >25 mm in women
- Reported or observed dysfunctional eating pattern
- Pairing food with other activities
- Concentrating food intake at the end of the day
- Eating in response to internal or external cues
- Sedentary activity level

Patient Outcomes
The patient will
- acknowledge the benefits of a healthy diet.
- develop and adhere to a healthy eating plan.
- avoid excessive alcohol intake.
- acknowledge the benefits of regular exercise.
- adopt and adhere to a regular exercise program.

Nursing Interventions	Rationales
Ask patient to maintain a food diary for several days and then discuss current eating habits with patient. Avoid making judgments.	This information provides a starting point for instruction as it clarifies which eating habits need modification and alteration.
Discuss with patient the correlation between food intake and weight and between weight and high blood pressure.	Overeating of carbohydrates and fats stimulates the sympathetic nervous system, which in turn increases heart rate and raises blood pressure. Overeating causes the pancreas to increase insulin levels to burn the extra calories. In Type II diabetes the tissues are resistant to the action of insulin, and in this case, the body also responds by producing additional insulin to maintain normal insulin activity. Increased circulating insulin levels are considered a major risk factor for development of cardiovascular disease in general and hypertension in particular.

Nursing Interventions	Rationales
Explain the need to avoid fats, oils, salt, and simple sugars in the diet and the importance of consuming recommended daily allowances of potassium, calcium, and magnesium. Instruct on portions and portion control. Avoid placing emphasis on calorie counting and the loss of a specific number of pounds per week.	Knowledge increases compliance. If the patient understands basic food composition, learns to omit these foods from the diet, and consumes appropriate portions of other foods, weight loss should occur. Counting calories can be frustrating and the stress of setting weight loss goals can destroy motivation.
Provide with choices upon which an eating plan can be developed by the patient. Place emphasis on the foods the patient can have.	Having choices reduces the feeling of deprivation.
Teach patient to interpret labels when grocery shopping.	Legislation has restricted unfounded claims on foods (for example, labeling vegetable oil "cholesterol free" even though it is still 100% fat). Labels are more comprehensive concerning amounts of nutrients. Patients may not understand the label and may not be able to apply the information to their specific diets, making instruction necessary. Canned foods may be nourishing but generally contain large amounts of sodium. Packaged foods frequently contain large amounts of fat, cholesterol, and sodium.
Teach patient healthy cooking methods.	Many healthy foods are rendered unhealthy due to cooking methods. Steaming and broiling avoids the need for additional fats in the diet.
Instruct patient to continue with food diary and discuss it with patient periodically. Weigh once a week. Praise and encourage patient for effort.	Maintaining the food diary reinforces the need for healthy food intake.
Advise patient to restrict alcohol intake to two drinks per day: 2 oz liquor, or 8 oz wine, or 24 oz beer.	Alcohol is a risk factor for hypertension.

Nursing Interventions	Rationales
Discuss the benefits of exercise and the correlation of exercise to hypertension.	Opioids normally inhibit blood pressure reaction to stress. Research indicates that certain brain nuclei do not secrete enough opioids to keep blood pressure in check during stressful situations in some people during the early stages of hypertension. Endurance exercise training may stimulate the brain to produce more opioids and thus reduce the blood pressure stress response. The National Institutes of Health recommend regular aerobic exercise (30–45 min brisk walk) three to five times per week. Aerobic exercise increases cardiovascular fitness and burns calories.
Question patient regarding choices for exercise: alone or in a group, indoors or outdoors. Consider other health problems that influence choices such as joint disease and cardiac or pulmonary disease. Videos are available for older adults and for exercises that are effective but carried out while sitting. Teach patient how to count pulse and determine target heart rate for walking programs or other exercise with aerobic benefits. Investigate other medications taken by patient.	Making choices gives the patient control of the situation. Working toward target heart rate can reinforce patient's knowledge of benefits of exercise. Some medications such as beta blockers can diminish exercise tolerance and affect target heart rate.
Help patient establish a plan so that a routine may be established.	If the patient selects the type of exercise and the time to do it, a routine is more quickly established and is more likely to be adhered to.

▶ NURSING DIAGNOSIS: *Anxiety (Chronic)*

Related To perceptions of stressful situations and inability to cope with stressful situations.

Defining Characteristics

Verbalization of

- apprehension
- uncertainty as to how to respond to situations
- fearfulness
- distress

Patient Outcomes

The patient will

- verbalize knowledge of relationship of stress to hypertension.
- verbalize useful measures for reducing stressful feelings.
- demonstrate ability to reduce stressful feelings.

Nursing Interventions	Rationales
Question patient regarding situations that produce stress reactions and how the reactions are managed.	Research proposes a link between individuals with type A personality traits and high blood pressure. Persons exhibiting type A traits may have ineffective stress responses.
Discuss with patient the relationship of stress to hypertension. Refer patient to effective stress management programs.	Research indicates that how an individual reacts to stress appears to be the key to whether hypertension develops (see rationale regarding opioid production above).
Explain the benefits of physical exercise for stress reduction. Provide resources for exercise training.	Exercise plus behavioral training in stress reduction techniques may lower blood pressure, thus avoiding, delaying, or reducing the dosage of antihypertensive medications.
Discuss coping mechanisms that have been used in the past. Reinforce need to continue with effective coping mechanisms.	Knowledge of past behaviors provides a starting point for further instruction. Coping mechanisms used in the past may or may not be effective.
Discuss situations that cause/increase anxiety.	Correlations can be made between situations and anxiety.
Provide resources for learning relaxation techniques: progressive relaxation, meditation, deep breathing, or guided imagery.	Research indicates that any of these techniques can be effective in stress reduction.

Nursing Interventions	Rationales
Teach problem-solving techniques: identification of problems, considering alternative solutions, possible outcomes for solutions, and selection of a solution.	This approach places the patient in control of the situation.

▶ NURSING DIAGNOSIS: *Knowledge Deficit (Medications)*

Related To lack of exposure to information regarding medications.

Defining Characteristics
Verbalization of lack of knowledge regarding medications

Patient Outcomes
The patient will
• verbalize knowledge of medications regarding
  −actions of medications
  −side effects
  −dosage
  −times of administration
  −necessity for taking medications as ordered
  −when and who to notify if side effects occur
• verbalize knowledge of need for frequent blood pressure checks as recommended.

Nursing Interventions	Rationales
Assess understanding of hypertension and previous teaching in regard to weight loss, diet, exercise. Identify misconceptions of health-related state.	Compliance with medication regime is more likely if patient has understanding of total treatment plan for hypertension management. The patient needs to be free of misconceptions before learning can occur.
Assess ability to learn and for deficits that can affect learning (see Patient Teaching, Appendix C, page 345).	The teaching/learning process has to be adapted to the individual needs of the patient. Elderly patients frequently have hearing and visual impairments. Include the family in the teaching program.

Nursing Interventions	Rationales
Check for accurate feedback.	Feedback provides for evaluation of learning, teaching, need for clarification, and reinforcement.
Reinforce teaching as necessary.	Repetition strengthens learning. Utilize various approaches to learning.

▶ **NURSING DIAGNOSIS:** *High Risk for Injury (Falling)*

Risk Factors
- Orthostatic hypotension
- Postprandial hypotension

Patient Outcomes
The patient will have decreased risk of falling due to orthostatic and postprandial hypotension.

Nursing Interventions	Rationales
Measure standing blood pressure.	Older persons are at risk of orthostatic hypotension, and drug dosages may need to be adjusted. Orthostatic hypotension is a frequent cause of falls in the elderly.
Instruct patient to remain seated on edge of bed before coming to standing position.	Standing too quickly causes a rapid fall in blood pressure when there is a change from a sitting or lying position to a standing position.
Measure blood pressure 30–60 min after eating.	Calcitonin gene–related peptide is a vasodilatory hormone that is released into circulation following eating. This is strongly correlated with a drop in blood pressure after meals, particularly for persons with systolic hypertension. Research indicates that an increase in falls in long-term care facilities occurs following meals.

Nursing Interventions	Rationales
Adjust the meal plan if postprandial hypotension is identified by decreasing the amount eaten at meals and increasing the frequency of meals. Unless contraindicated, increase fat content.	Postprandial hypotension is related to the carbohydrate content of the meal. The risk is greater after a glucose load.

▶ **NURSING DIAGNOSIS:** *Noncompliance (Smoking)*

Related To
• Smoking as a coping mechanism
• Previous unsuccessful attempts to quit smoking
• Denial of present health problems

Defining Characteristics
• Observed smoking
• Reports of family
• Self-reports of smoking

Patient Outcomes
The patient will
• acknowledge need for smoking cessation.
• identify personal reasons for smoking and develop plans to deal with cues for smoking.
• set target date for smoking cessation.
• stop smoking.
• utilize effective coping techniques to deal with withdrawal symptoms.

Nursing Interventions	Rationales
Teach the consequences of smoking.	There is a direct correlation between smoking and hypertension. The consequences of hypertension include cardiac disease and stroke. Smoking also increases the risk of pulmonary disease and cancer of the bladder and pancreas. Passive smoking is dangerous to nonsmokers. Smoking is expensive.

Nursing Interventions	Rationales
Identify cues which prompt smoking.	There are specific times and situations which trigger a need for smoking, i.e., after a meal, while watching television. After identifying these cues, management techniques can be implemented to avoid smoking.
Help to develop a specific plan to stop smoking. Provide information on community programs and discuss individual techniques for smoking cessation.	The probability of success is greater when the patient can choose the method.
Teach short- and long-term methods to cope with withdrawal symptoms.	Chewing gum or sugar-free candy, oral hygiene, drinking a glass of water, distraction, and moving about are effective short-term techniques. Long-term techniques include stress reduction methods (see page 90, anxiety) and exercise.

DISCHARGE PLANNING/CONTINUITY OF CARE
- Evaluate knowledge of hypertension and life-style modifications.
- Reinforce need for regular follow-up care.
- Provide information for smoking cessation classes if necessary.
- Provide information for weight control classes if necessary.
- Arrange for consultation with dietician.
- Reinforce information regarding medications and the importance of compliance with medication regime.

Clinical Clip

- Systolic and diastolic blood pressures tend to rise with age. After age 50, diastolic pressure levels off but systolic pressure may continue to increase, leading to isolated systolic hypertension (ISH), defined as a systolic blood pressure of 140 mm Hg or more with diastolic blood pressure below 90 mm Hg. In middle-aged and older people ISH is a more accurate predictor for cardiovascular morbidity and mortality than diastolic pressure.

- Pseudohypertension in the elderly is due to rigid brachial arteries. To rule out this possibility, palpate the radial artery when the sphygmomanometer is fully inflated. If the artery is still palpable, it is likely that the high reading is due to a rigid brachial artery.

BIBLIOGRAPHY

American Heart Association. (1990/91). Brain "control centers" link stress to high blood pressure. *Heartstyle, 1*(2), 7.

American Heart Association. (1991). Insulin elevation may be a major risk factor for high blood pressure. *Heartstyle, 1*(3), 7.

American Heart Association. (1991/92). Behavior and blood pressure—when an "A" may be an F. *Heartstyle, 2*(1), 2.

American Heart Association. (1989/90). INTERSALT study of 52 groups confirms link between salt and high blood pressure. *Cardiovascular Research Report, 33*, 2.

Johannsen, J. (1993). UPDATE: Guidelines for treating hypertension. *American Journal of Nursing, 93*(3), 42–49.

Lenfant, C. (1992). Controlling high blood pressure and preventing strokes. *Be Stroke Smart, 9*(2), 3–4.

Morley, J. E. (1993). The ultimate Big Mac attack. *Nursing Home Medicine, 1*(4), 3.

Reducing the health consequences of smoking: 25 years of progress. (1989). A Report of the Surgeon General. U.S. Department of Health and Human Services. Bethesda, MD.

Trottier, D. J., & Kochar, M. S. (1993). Managing isolated systolic hypertension. *American Journal of Nursing, 93*(10), 50–53.

PERIPHERAL VASCULAR DISEASE: LOWER EXTREMITIES

The term peripheral vascular disease (PVD) refers to pathology of any blood vessels (arteries or veins) and lymphatics away from the heart. Blood flow is diminished and, without intervention, can lead to ischemic pain, skin ulcerations, gangrene, and amputation.

ETIOLOGIES
- Arterial
  - arterial occlusive disease due to atherosclerotic plaque
  - aneurysm
  - vasospasms
  - arteritis
  - compartment or compression syndrome
- Venous
  - thrombus
  - thrombophlebitis
  - incompetent venous valves

CLINICAL MANIFESTATIONS
- Arterial
  - skin pale on elevation, becomes dusky red on dependency
  - skin thin, shiny, atrophic
  - hair loss over feet and toes
  - toenails thick and rigid
  - ulcers
  - cool skin temperature
  - loss of arterial pulsations
  - burning pain during exercise

–intermittent claudication
–bruits present if artery is obstructed
- Venous
  –cyanosis on dependency
  –petechiae, brown pigmentation
  –ulcers if present, noted on sides of ankles
  –normal skin temperature unless phlebitis is present, causing warmth
  –chronic edema
  –distended, tortuous veins
  –feeling of heaviness in extremities after prolonged standing

CLINICAL/DIAGNOSTIC FINDINGS
- Arterial
  –Doppler ultrasound: diminished sound waves if arterial occlusion or stenosis
  –plethysmography: reduced blood volume changes
  –pressure measurement: drop in pressure in area of stenosis or occlusion
  –stress testing: flattened waveform, drop in ankle pressure
  –arteriography: occlusive disease, arterial emboli, trauma, aneurysm
  –computerized (CT) scan: abdominal aortic aneurysms, postoperative complications
- Venous
  –Doppler ultrasound: changes in sound wave frequency
  –plethysmography: decreased flow
  –ambulatory venous pressure measurement: diminished pressure drop with exercise, recovery time less than 20 s
  –manual compression: incompetent valves
  –retrograde filling test: incompetent valves
  –magnetic resonance imaging (MRI): deep-vein thrombosis
  –venography: venous abnormalities
  –B/mode venous imaging: disruptions of flow, thrombus, valvular incompetency

▶ NURSING DIAGNOSIS: *Altered Peripheral Tissue Perfusion*

Related To PVD.

Defining Characteristics
(See Clinical Manifestations)

Patient Outcomes
The patient will
- verbalize knowledge of disease, treatment, actions, and side effects of medications.
- alter life-style as indicated by causative factors.

- remain free of skin/tissue impairments in affected extremities.
- verbalize knowledge of prevention and signs of complications.

Nursing Interventions	Rationales
Assess lower extremities for the following: 1. skin texture, color, edema, ulcerations, hair loss over feet/toes 2. capillary refill 3. presence/rate, rhythm, and quality of pulses bilaterally and simultaneously/auscultate over pulse points if obstruction is suspected 4. pain: when it occurs and precipitating factors 5. calf tenderness (Homan's sign)	The assessment will differentiate between arterial and venous disease.
Assess mental status.	Persons with PVD are also at risk for cerebral vascular disease, which can cause confusion and disorientation.
Prepare patient and provide instructions for diagnostic tests.	Patient must be knowledgeable enough to give informed consent, particularly for invasive procedures such as arteriography.
Instruct patient on the disease, the treatment, actions, and side effects of medications. Evaluate factors in life-style that may aggravate or advance atherosclerosis: smoking, obesity, hyperlipidemia, hypertension, diabetes.	The informed patient has a decreased risk of noncompliance. Interventions can be implemented for smoking cessation programs, weight loss programs, increased stress levels, and nutritional instruction to reduce levels of blood lipids. Further evaluation of chronic diseases such as hypertension and diabetes may reveal a need for additional treatment.
Instruct patients with chronic venous insufficiency to 1. elevate the legs while in bed and periodically throughout the day. 2. wear graduated compression stockings whenever out of bed	Venous flow of blood is facilitated. The extremity becomes edematous in the dependent position and recedes when the extremity is elevated. If it does not, the edema is unrelated to the venous circulation.

Nursing Interventions	Rationales
and to put stockings on before getting out of bed. 3. avoid prolonged sitting or standing by moving around at least every hour. 4. lose weight if obese. Instruct all patients to avoid 5. wearing round garters. 6. crossing the legs while sitting.	Round garters and crossing the legs constrict circulation.
Teach patient and family Buerger-Allen exercises: 1. Lie flat with feet elevated above heart level for about 2 min or until blanching occurs. 2. Now dangle on the edge of the bed and move feet around for about 5 min or until the legs turn pink. 3. Lie flat with legs flat for 5 min. 4. Repeat the sequence five times and do exercises three times a day.	This exercise encourages circulation.
Instruct patient on signs of thrombosis.	Thrombosis is a possible complication associated with PVD.
Instruct patient on foot care and inspection (see Diabetes Mellitus, page 193).	Elderly individuals are at risk for impaired skin and tissue integrity because of aging changes that cause the skin to be more fragile. Elderly persons with PVD have an additional risk for skin impairment, vascular ulcers, infection, and gangrene due to the disruptions in blood flow and resulting ischemia. Any trauma including the smallest break in the skin can lead to ulceration and possibly eventual amputation. Every effort should be made to teach the patient the necessity for taking meticulous care of the feet and for completing

Nursing Interventions	Rationales
	thorough inspections of the feet on a regular basis. Following a scrupulous routine will help to prevent these complications.

▶ NURSING DIAGNOSIS: *Pain (May Be Acute or Chronic When Related to Arterial Disease)*

Related To ischemia of tissue due to disruptions in blood flow.

Defining Characteristics
- Acute pain related to arterial disease: sudden onset, constant pain not relieved by rest or activity (usually results from acute embolic occlusion of artery)
- Chronic pain related to arterial disease
  - intermittent claudication (burning, fatigue, ache, cramping) during exercise and subsides within a few minutes with rest
  - rest pain: burning pain occurring soon after lying flat in bed (usually results from severe arterial occlusion)
- Pain related to venous disease
  - generally no pain unless thrombophlebitis is present causing pain along the course of the vein
  - venous claudication (acute, intense onset of cramping in calf after prolonged standing or exercise)

Patient Outcomes
The patient will
- report pain when it occurs.
- recognize pain that requires immediate intervention by physician (pain resulting from occlusions).
- verbalize knowledge of pain-relieving measures.
- verbalize decrease in level of pain.

Nursing Interventions	Rationales
Assess the pain: 1. type of onset 2. when it occurs 3. relationship to rest, exercise	An accurate pain assessment can provide abundant information: 1. Rule out neurological or ortho- pedic causes of pain.

Nursing Interventions	Rationales
4. area of extremity that is affected 5. nature of pain: acute, chronic, sharp, dull, aching	2. Determine whether pain is due to arterial or venous insufficiency; both forms of PVD may be present in the same person. 3. Location of pain indicates the vessels involved. 4. Burning pain and numbness at night signal disease progression to peripheral nerve ischemia. 5. Severe, constant arterial pain can result in functional deficits and lead to complete ischemia, gangrene, and amputation.
Teach/assist to position extremity for comfort: 1. Arterial rest pain: Place foot in dependent position. 2. Venous pain: Elevate extremity above level of heart. 3. Avoid using knee gatch or pillows under knees.	Pain in horizontal position indicates failure of collateral vessels to perfuse adequately. Lowering the extremity will increase blood flow. Elevating extremity promotes venous drainage. Pressure under knee constricts circulation.
Maintain warmth of extremity. 1. Maintain room temperature between 72 and 74 F. 2. Instruct to wear wool or cotton socks when walking or in bed. 3. Avoid external sources of heat, i.e., heating pads.	Maintaining warmth increases vasodilation, improving blood flow, thus relieving pain due to ischemia. Ischemic tissue is at risk for injury from external sources of heat.
Place sheepskin under lower extremities. Place lambswool between the toes. Keep linens off the toes. Apply heel protectors or floating heels.	These measures reduce discomfort related to pressure, friction, and trauma.
Administer analgesics as prescribed and monitor effectiveness.	Use of extremity can be encouraged when comfort level is increased.
Instruct to establish a routine walking program: 1. Arterial disease: Walk until cramping or pain begins, then	Walking helps develop arterial collateral circulation to bypass blocked artery. Venous drainage is increased.

Nursing Interventions

rest; when pain subsides, try to walk further, gradually increasing distance.
2. Venous disease: Walk every hour and at least once a day; walk as long as condition permits; elevate legs afterward.

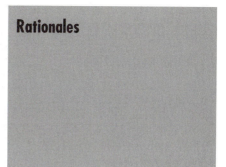

▶ **NURSING DIAGNOSIS:** *Impaired Tissue Integrity*

Related To altered circulation.

Defining Characteristics
* Damaged integument and subcutaneous tissue
* Arterial ulcers
  –located on toes or other pressure points of foot
  –often symmetrical
  –drainage usually not present
* Venous ulcers: located on ankle, usually medially

Patient Outcomes
The patient will
* remain free of infection.
* provide evidence of tissue regeneration.
* maintain adequate nutritional status.

Nursing Interventions	Rationales
Monitor for 1. new epithelial and granulation tissue, exudate, pus, and necrotic tissue. 2. factors contributing to delayed healing: redness, edema, and bruising around ulcer.	Monitoring helps to determine whether present treatment is effective and identifies infection promptly for appropriate treatment.
Continue with interventions to increase peripheral circulation.	Any decrease in peripheral circulation will exacerbate the disease and retard healing of ulcers if present.

Nursing Interventions	Rationales
Assess nutritional status.	Altered nutritional status may prolong/prevent healing.
Maintain ulcer in appropriate physiological environment: 1. Maintain cleanliness with irrigation, removing debris and exudate. 2. Debride necrotic tissue with autolysis, enzymes, surgical excision, or wet-to-damp dressings. 3. Select treatment that provides moist environment and establish schedule congruent with treatment method. (See Pressure Ulcer, page 22.)	

DISCHARGE PLANNING/CONTINUITY OF CARE
- Evaluate patient's knowledge regarding medications and treatment regime.
- Provide instructions for follow-up monitoring and care with primary care provider.
- Instruct and encourage to continue with life-style changes involving diet, smoking, exercise, and stress management.
- Provide information for consultation or classes for diet, smoking cessation, exercise, and stress management if necessary.
- Arrange for home health nurse to monitor and provide treatment for ulcers if present.

--- Clinical Clip ---

Research indicates that distal bypass is often a viable alternative to amputation for persons with PVD. If preoperative evaluation clears the patient over 75 for surgery, the risk for complications is no higher than for patients under 75. Balloon angioplasty may be the treatment of choice if the narrowing of the vessel is below 6 cm and localized.

BIBLIOGRAPHY
Bright, L. D., & Georgi, S. (1992). Peripheral vascular disease—Is it arterial or venous? *American Journal of Nursing, 92*(11), 34–43.

Cameron, J., et al. (1992). Contact dermatitis in leg ulcer patients. *Ostomy/Wound Management, 38*(9), 8–11.

Eliopoulos, C. (1991). P.V.D. Protecting patients from complications. *Nursing 91, 21*(4), 32c, 32f.

Gogia, P. P. (1992). The biology of wound healing. *Ostomy/Wound Management, 38*(9), 12, 14–16, 18–20, 22.

Kuhn, J. K., & McGovern, M. (1992). Peripheral vascular assessment of the elderly client. *Journal of Gerontological Nursing, 18*(12), 35–38.

Stotts, N. (1993). Wound care practices in the United States. *Ostomy/Wound Management, 39*(3), 28–34.

$\mathcal{T}$RANSIENT ISCHEMIC ATTACK

Transient ischemic attacks (TIAs) are momentary episodes of focal loss of brain function. These attacks are rapid in onset and generally last 2–15 min but may last as long as 24 h. The longer the attack, the greater the likelihood that a cerebral infarct is present. Symptoms are similar to those of stroke but are reversible and temporary. There are two types of TIA: vertebrobasilar and carotid. Transient ischemic attacks may occur once or several times in a lifetime. Persons experiencing TIAs are at risk for eventually suffering a stroke.

ETIOLOGIES
- Elevated cholesterol levels (when cholesterol levels are high, the platelets secrete increased amounts of chemicals that constrict blood vessels, leading to artery spasms and resulting in TIA)

CLINICAL MANIFESTATIONS
- Vertebrobasilar TIA
  - hemiparesis or hemiplegia of any combination of upper and lower extremities and face, left and/or right
  - paresthesia involving left, right, or both sides
  - diplopia or blurred vision
  - partial or total blindness
  - dysarthria
  - aphasia
  - dysphagia
- Carotid TIA
  - hemiparesis or hemiplegia
  - homonymous hemianopsia
  - paresthesia of right upper extremity and/or lower extremity and/or face
  - aphasia
  - dysarthria

107

CLINICAL/DIAGNOSTIC FINDINGS

- Based on history
- Findings suggestive of vessel disease (may be present in absence of history of TIAs)
  - bruit over carotid artery
  - emboli in retinal vessels
  - difference of >15 mm Hg between systolic pressures of arms
- Diagnostic tests (findings of cerebral vascular dysfunction)
  - computerized tomography (CT) scan
  - magnetic resonance imaging (MRI)
  - cerebral angiography
  - carotid Doppler studies
- Differential diagnosis includes migraine, seizures, Meniere's syndrome, hypotensive syncope, hypoglycemia, and narcolepsy

▶ NURSING DIAGNOSIS: *Altered Tissue Perfusion (Cerebral)*

Related To disease of cerebral blood vessels.

Defining Characteristics
(See Clinical Manifestations)

Patient Outcomes
The patient will alter life-style in an attempt to reduce risk factors associated with stroke.

Nursing Interventions	Rationales
Assess current knowledge of disease process. Explain relationship between risk factors, TIA, and stroke. Plan a teaching program to assist in reducing risk factors: 1. smoking 2. obesity 3. hypertension 4. lack of exercise 5. high-fat, high-cholesterol, high-sodium diet	The patient must be knowledgeable in order to be compliant with health care regime.
Assess nutritional status. If patient is overweight, advise weight reduction management plan. Provide instructions for reducing sodium	Obesity is a risk factor for stroke. Loss of weight reduces this risk. High cholesterol is associated with vessel disease that causes TIA.

Nursing Interventions	Rationales
and cholesterol intake. (See Hypertension, page 88.)	High sodium intake is related to hypertension.
Question patient concerning use of tobacco. Advise a smoking cessation program. (See Hypertension, page 94.)	Smoking increases the risk of stroke. Research confirms a correlation between long-term cigarette use, the density of fatty plaque obstructing cerebral arteries, and the likelihood of stroke.
Assist in planning exercise program (see Hypertension, page 90).	Regular aerobic exercise conditions cardiovascular function and increases blood flow to brain.
Provide information on prescribed medications: dosage, administration times, actions, and side effects.	Antiplatelet agents (aspirin) and anticoagulants (coumadin or heparin) are frequently prescribed for TIA. Patient must be aware of potential for bleeding.
Instruct patient to have blood pressure checked regularly.	Hypertension is frequently associated with TIA and is a risk factor for stroke.

DISCHARGE PLANNING/CONTINUITY OF CARE
- Provide for appropriate consultations if patient has difficulty maintaining recommended life-style changes.
- Arrange for follow-up blood pressure checks.
- Instruct patient to call primary care provider if TIA symptoms recur.

BIBLIOGRAPHY
American Heart Association. (1992). High cholesterol may signal warning for potential stroke. *Heartstyle, 2*(2), 8.

American Heart Association. (1992). Avoiding a stroke. *American Heart News, 9*(2), 6–7.

American Heart Association. (1989/90). TIA is stroke early warning signal. *Cardiovascular Research Report, 33*, 3.

Kane-Carlsen, P. A. (1992). Managing patients with TIAs. *Nursing 92, 22*(1), 34–39.

National Institute of Neurological Disorders and Stroke. (1989). *Classification of cerebrovascular diseases III*. Bethesda, MD: National Institutes of Health.

Pulmonary
Conditions

CHRONIC OBSTRUCTIVE PULMONARY DISEASE

While one disease may predominate, chronic obstructive pulmonary disease (COPD) is a combination of two closely related conditions: emphysema and chronic bronchitis. Chronic bronchitis is defined as a cough and expectoration that lasts at least 3 months out of the year for 2 consecutive years or for 6 months during 1 year. With emphysema, the alveoli of the lungs are damaged and enlarged. This reduces the surface area for the exchange of oxygen and carbon dioxide. The COPD is characterized by airway obstruction, air trapping, and hypoxemia. It is progressive, irreversible, and degenerative, causing only minimal disability in some people but overwhelming respiratory distress in others.

ETIOLOGIES
- Emphysema: an imbalance between a lung protease (elastase) and alpha-1-protease inhibitor causing destruction of alveolar walls and bronchioles; in majority of cases, imbalance due to smoking
- Chronic bronchitis: smoking and inhaling environmental irritants and severe, recurrent infections

CLINICAL MANIFESTATIONS
- Chronic cough (productive during periods of infection)
- Shortness of breath
- Frequent respiratory tract infections

CLINICAL/DIAGNOSTIC FINDINGS
- Clinical laboratory tests
  - Alpha-1-antitrypsin determination: normal values, >250 mg/dL; deficient or absent serum levels indicate early onset of emphysema
- Radiologic tests
  - Chest x-ray: deviations from normal may indicate COPD
- Nuclear scanning tests

–Lung scan: deviations from normal may indicate emphysema
- Pulmonary function studies

NOTE: Normal values vary with age, sex, height, and weight. Values less than 50% of the expected norm indicate poor pulmonary function.

–forced vital capacity (FVC)
–forced expiratory volume in 1 s (FEV_1)
–maximal midexpiratory flow rate (MMEF)
–maximal voluntary ventilation (MVV)

▶ NURSING DIAGNOSIS: *Ineffective Breathing Pattern*

Related To obstruction of airflow during exhalation.

Defining Characteristics
- Dyspnea
- Shortness of breath
- Cough
- Nasal flaring
- Use of accessory muscles for breathing
- Changes in respiratory depth

Patient Outcomes
The patient will
- display self-help techniques by utilizing effective breathing techniques.
- experience effective breathing patterns evidenced by decreased respiratory rates during physical activity.
- utilize metered-dose inhaler or nebulizer effectively as prescribed.
- exhibit decreased anxiety caused from ineffective breathing patterns.

Nursing Interventions	Rationales
Elevate the head of the bed to a position of comfort. Tell the patient to let the shoulders relax and place pillows under the elbows.	Lungs expand more easily and shoulder strain is avoided.
Teach patient to use pursed-lip breathing when short of breath: 1. Sit upright with hands on thighs and lean forward with elbows propped on a table. 2. Breathe in slowly through the nose with mouth closed. 3. Purse lips as though whistling and breathe the air out through	Pursed-lip breathing allows more oxygenated air to be inhaled and maintains the patency of the airway during expiration, which helps empty the lungs and slow down the respiratory rate.

Nursing Interventions	**Rationales**
the mouth slowly and evenly, without forcing it. 4. Contract abdominal muscles while breathing out. Exhalation should take at least twice as long as inhalation.	
Teach diaphragmatic breathing after patient feels comfortable with pursed-lip breathing: Have the patient practice while lying down or sitting up and then while walking. As the exercise becomes easier, it can be performed with any activity. 1. Have the patient place one hand below the ribs, over the abdomen and the other on the middle of the chest. 2. Push abdomen out against hand while inhaling slowly through nose. 3. Exhale through pursed lips to the count of 3 while tightening abdominal muscles. 4. When walking, count with steps and take two steps for inspiration and three to four steps for expiration.	This increases the ability to breathe deeply into the lungs. Expiration is prolonged, thereby decreasing respiratory rate. Abdominal muscles are strengthened so they can assist with breathing and the diaphragm is used instead of the accessory muscles.
Teach patient to 1. prepare medications for inhaler. 2. administer medications through the inhaler. 3. recognize signs of side effects from medications. 4. clean and disinfect equipment (see Table 13.1, page 121).	The medication is ineffective if not prepared and administered correctly. Appropriate cleaning and disinfecting prevents bacterial growth.
Teach patient and caregiver to monitor for signs and symptoms of cor pulmonale: 1. increase in coughing, dyspnea, and fatigue 2. peripheral edema 3. sudden weight gain	Cor pulmonale is a complication of COPD. The right ventricle enlarges, causing pulmonary hypertension, resulting in hypoxia and acidosis. The condition may be acute or chronic and needs immediate attention.

▶ NURSING DIAGNOSIS: *Ineffective Airway Clearance*

Related To ineffective cough and inability to remove airway secretions.

Defining Characteristics
- Abnormal breath sounds: rales, rhonchi
- Changes in rate or depth of respiration
- Ineffective cough
- Dyspnea

Patient Outcomes
The patient will demonstrate ability to remove airway secretions by coughing effectively.

Nursing Interventions	Rationales
Teach the patient to cough and clear the airway: 1. Explain that the best time to use coughing techniques is upon arising in the morning. Avoid coughing on a full stomach because it may cause vomiting. 2. Instruct patient to sit upright with head slightly forward and feet on the floor. Do pursed-lip breathing once or twice. 3. Breathe in again but only to the midinspiratory point, hold the breath for a few seconds, and then cough twice in rapid succession: once to loosen the mucus and the second time to bring it up. Remind patient not to take any quick breaths between coughs. 4. Advise patient to use this procedure with coughing.	Coughing spells can cause fatigue and anxiety, increasing respiratory distress. The increased mucus production, loss of lung elasticity, and narrowed bronchial airways prevent an effective cough. Learning to control the cough (not suppress it) and to cough deeply will allow enough air pressure to move mucus from the lungs and to clear the airway.
Administer chest physical therapy if prescribed by physician: postural drainage, percussion, and vibration. Chest physical therapy is only performed 1. after a thorough evaluation of respiratory and cardiovascular status.	Postural drainage utilizes the force of gravity in removing retained secretions from the bronchioles. Coughing facilitates the movement of the secretions into the bronchi and trachea for expectoration. Percussion and

Nursing Interventions	Rationales
2. if there are secretions present in the lungs. 3. by trained personnel.	vibration dislodges thick, tenacious secretions from the bronchial walls.
Maintain a fluid intake of 2,500 mL/day. Warm, clear liquids are preferable. Avoid beverages containing caffeine or alcohol. Milk should be avoided if it thickens the mucus.	Adequate fluid intake liquifies chest secretions, making it easier to clear the secretions from the lungs.
Monitor for signs of congestive heart failure: rales, edema, and weight gain. Measure and record intake and output.	Increased fluid intake presents risk of congestive heart failure.
Give expectorants or bronchodilators as prescribed.	These loosen and facilitate expectoration of secretions.

▶ NURSING DIAGNOSIS: *Activity Intolerance*

Related To shortness of breath with exertion.

Defining Characteristics
- Complains of shortness of breath with exertion
- Respirations increased and gasping

Patient Outcomes
The patient will
- ambulate two times each day.
- give evidence of increasing strength and endurance by walking longer distances without increased respiratory distress.
- maintain breathing and pulse rates within acceptable parameters.
- participate in the exercise plan twice each day.

Nursing Interventions	Rationales
Set up a schedule for ambulation twice a day and gradually increase the distance.	Daily exercise helps alleviate complications associated with inactivity. Walking every day increases strength and endurance.
Accompany patient on walks, reminding to count steps with two	Walking with the patient offers opportunity for monitoring the

Nursing Interventions	Rationales
steps for inspiration and four for expiration. Reinforce breathing techniques while walking. Provide encouragement and praise.	patient's condition and ability to utilize appropriate breathing techniques.
Monitor breathing and pulse rate. Administer supplemental oxygen at 1–3 LPM if necessary during periods of increased activity (see Table 13.2, page 121).	Without adequate activity, large muscles become deconditioned and consume more oxygen, placing an additional burden on the lungs. If administered at excessive levels, O_2 can cause diminished hypoxic drive in patients who chronically retain carbon dioxide (CO_2). This results in CO_2 narcosis and respiratory failure.
Carry out active assistive range-of-motion (ROM) exercises twice a day. As strength increases, have patient do active exercises. Add stretching activities to the routine as endurance improves.	The ROM exercises maintain joint flexibility. Active assistive ROM (AAROM) and active ROM (AROM) provide minimal aerobic affects.
Transport per wheelchair for long distances.	Using the wheelchair broadens the patient's scope of socialization.

▶ **NURSING DIAGNOSIS:** *High Risk for Infection (Respiratory Tract)*

Risk Factors
- Inadequate ventilation due to COPD
- Insufficient fluid intake
- Physical inactivity
- Compromised defenses

Patient Outcomes
The patient will remain free of respiratory tract infections.

Nursing Interventions	Rationales
Monitor for signs of infection: 1. fever 2. increased pulse rate 3. increased shortness of breath 4. changes in the amount, consistency, and color of mucus 5. loss of appetite	Prompt identification of infection allows for prompt treatment.
Monitor for periods of agitation or disorientation. Report changes to the physician promptly.	Older people do not always have elevated temperatures or other classical signs of infection. Cognitive changes may be the only indication of physical changes.
Consult with the physician for administration of influenza and pneumonia vaccine.	Vaccines decrease the risk of respiratory tract infection. In the elderly patient, pneumonia is frequently preceded by influenza.
Advise patient to 1. restrict outdoor activities during periods of increased air pollution and during hot and cold weather. 2. avoid tobacco smoke. 3. avoid close contact with persons who have respiratory tract infections. 4. stay away from areas where paint or other fumes are present. 5. eliminate the use of perfumed lotions and bath powders.	Irritation of the lungs from external sources increases the risk of respiratory infection.
Disinfect or sterilize inhalation devices at least daily or as the manufacturer directs.	Disinfection/sterilization avoids the transfer of microorganisms to the respiratory tract by indirect contact.

▶ NURSING DIAGNOSIS: *Fear*

Related To shortness of breath secondary to COPD.

Defining Characteristics

Verbalizes feelings of panic when short of breath.

Patient Outcomes

The patient will verbalize a feeling of control by utilizing breathing exercises.

Nursing Interventions	Rationales
Teach relaxation techniques that can be combined with pursed-lip breathing to relieve tension: 1. Have patient sit in a quiet room in a comfortable chair with arms and legs supported and eyes closed. 2. Do pursed-lip breathing and, during exhalation, imagine breathing the tension out of the body. 3. Tighten various sets of muscles and then relax them. Start with the forehead and face and neck muscles and progress down the body by shrugging shoulders, tightening arm muscles, and making fists. 4. After tensing each part, relax the muscles and do pursed-lip breathing before going on to the next part. 5. Imagine soft breezes, the roar of the ocean, or birds singing to aid in relaxation. Think "I am in control" while going through the exercises.	As the patient gains control of breathing by learning and using these procedures, anxiety and fear should decrease. The relaxation techniques will alleviate feelings of fright and apprehension.

DISCHARGE PLANNING/CONTINUITY OF CARE

For home discharge:
- Assess understanding of medications and when and how to take them.
- Assess ability to identify signs of infection and when to call the physician.
- Assess ability to use and clean breathing aids.
- Arrange for meals-on-wheels to ensure adequate nutrition if there is no significant other available to do this.
- Arrange for home health aid to assist with exercises and diversional activities.

Table 13.1 • Using An Inhaler

Inhalers are used to disperse medication through an aerosol mist, spray, or powder. The medication is administered to dilate narrowed bronchioles or to loosen thick mucus secretions. The drug is placed in a canister that fits into the inhaler. The inhaler is metered to deliver a specific amount of medication with each inhalation. The patient must learn how to use the equipment and to be aware of the hazards of overuse. These directions are written for the patient:

1. If more than one medication is to be taken by inhalation, administer the bronchodilator first. The second medication will then be fully inhaled.
2. Shake the canister.
3. Remove the protective cap.
4. Hold inhaler with your index finger on the top of the metal canister and your thumb on the bottom of the plastic mouthpiece.
5. Place the inhaler in your mouth, just past your front teeth. Direct the opening toward the back of your throat.
6. Empty the lungs by exhaling fully. Then grasp the mouthpiece with your teeth and lips.
7. Inhale slowly and deeply while you are depressing the medication canister. Breathing deeply carries the particles of medication deep into the lungs. It is important to inhale while the spray is administered.
8. Hold your breath for 10 s or as long as you are comfortable. The medicine will remain in your lungs when you exhale.
9. Exhale slowly through pursed lips.
10. Cough up the mucus.
11. Wait a few minutes between inhalations or as long as the directions indicate.
12. Rinse your mouth out with water when you are finished.
13. Replace protective cap back on inhaler.
14. Rinse mouthpiece and cap at least daily with warm water and dry thoroughly.
15. Systemic side effects of bronchodilators include shakiness, dizziness, sweating, irritability, insomnia, feelings of anxiety, and increased heart rate.

Table 13.2 • Oxygen Therapy

Nasal Cannula

1–6 LPM
Rate should not exceed 2 LPM for persons with COPD or the stimulus to breathe is depressed. This method is appropriate for mouth breathers.
Oxygen concentration cannot be controlled.
Keep humidifier jar filled.
Check flow rate and cannula frequently. Check nares for skin breakdown.

Table 13.2 • *continued*

Nasal Catheter

Not over 2–3 LPM for persons with COPD. Set flow rate before insertion.
Measure from patient's nose to earlobe for length of catheter to be inserted.
Lubricate with water-soluble jelly.
After insertion, catheter should be visible on either side of uvula; withdraw
so it is no longer visible.
Secure catheter to nose and cheek.
Change catheter every 8 h and reinsert in opposite nares.

Simple Mask

5–8 LPM
Oxygen concentration cannot be controlled.
Mask should fit snugly but should not press tightly against skin.

Non-Rebreathing Mask

6–15 LPM; delivers up to 90% oxygen
One-way valve separates nonrebreather mask from bag. Valve opens during
inhalation to allow oxygen to enter mask. One-way valve on mask closes to
prevent mixing of room air. During exhalation, valve between mask and
bag closes to prevent expired carbon dioxide from entering bag. Valves on
mask open to release exhaled carbon dioxide.
Make sure valves are secure and functioning.
Bag must remain inflated during both inspiration and expiration.
Marked or complete deflation indicates flow rate is too low.

Partial Rebreather Mask

6–15 LPM; delivers up to 60% oxygen
The partial rebreather mask does not have the one-way valve between reser-
voir bag and mask.

Aerosol Mask

Oxygen concentrations can be adjusted from 25 to 100%.
Use sterile water and remove condensed water from tubing at regular intervals.
Mist must be constantly available during inhalation.

Intermittent Positive Pressure Breathing

Machine is plugged into a pressure source: oxygen or compressed air.
Prescribed medication or saline is placed in nebulizer.
Machine is regulated to deliver pressure on inhalation assisting patient to
breathe deeply.
Controls are adjusted according to directions for machine or physician's
orders.
Patient must seal lips around mouthpiece and breathe only through mouth.

BIBLIOGRAPHY

Bolgiano, C. S., Bunting, K., & Shoenberger, N. M. (1990). Administering oxygen therapy: What you need to know. *Nursing 90, 20*(6), 47–51.

DaCunha, J. P. (Ed.). (1991). *Respiratory support.* Springhouse, PA: Springhouse Corporation.

Gyetvan, M. C., & McMann, J. A. S. (Eds.). (1988). *Diseases and disorders handbook.* Springhouse, PA: Springhouse Corporation.

Hickey, M. (1990). Controlling cor pulmonale. *Nursing 90, 20*(5), 32E, 32H.

Janelli, L. M., Scherer, Y. K., & Schmieder, L. E. (1991). Can a pulmonary health teaching program alter patients' ability to cope with COPD? *Rehabilitation Nursing, 16*(4), 199–202.

McCann, J. A. S. (1991). (Ed.). *Diagnostic test implications.* Springhouse, PA: Springhouse Corporation.

National Institutes of Health. (1986). *Chronic obstructive pulmonary disease.* Washington, DC: U.S. Department of Health and Human Services.

Schull, P. D. (1992). *Nursing procedures.* Springhouse, PA: Springhouse Corporation.

Swearingen, P. L. (1992). *Pocket guide to medical-surgical nursing.* St. Louis, MO: Mosby Year-Book.

$\mathcal{P}$NEUMONIA

Expected age-related changes of the respiratory system increase the risk of pneumonia among the elderly (see Aging Changes, Appendix A, page 338). Nutritional deficiencies, dehydration, altered mental status, functional deficits, and multiple medical diagnoses are predisposing factors. Frequently, the patient is diagnosed with primary influenza pneumonia and, after initial improvement, develops an exacerbation of signs and symptoms due to secondary bacterial pneumonia when the virus spreads to the alveolar epithelium. Aspiration pneumonia is also common. Gram negative bacteria are frequently found in the mouth and may cause pneumonia if aspirated.

ETIOLOGIES
- Primary influenza pneumonia: A or B virus
- Secondary bacterial pneumonia
  - *Streptococcus pneumoniae*
  - *Staphylococcus aureus*
  - *Haemophilus influenza*

CLINICAL MANIFESTATIONS
The signs and symptoms of pneumonia may be distorted by underlying conditions and by development of secondary problems such as congestive heart failure or respiratory failure. Two signs are most consistently associated with pneumonia in the elderly:
- tachypnea
- tachycardia

Other signs and symptoms may include the following:
- fever
- chills
- myalgia
- cough
- sputum production
- dyspnea
- pleuritic chest pain

NOTE: The signs and symptoms of acute illness are frequently blunted and atypical in older adults due to diminished immune responsiveness and reduced inflammatory response. These clinical manifestations require investigation as they frequently signal the onset of acute illness:

- alterations in mental status
- changes in usual activity pattern
- falling
- decreased food intake
- weight loss
- general deterioration

CLINICAL/DIAGNOSTIC FINDINGS

- Diffuse crackles found on auscultation
- Evidence of consolidation and pleural effusion by physical examination and chest x-ray
- Isolation of microorganism from sputum samples

NOTE: It is difficult to obtain sputum specimens from elderly patients, and medical management is frequently based on clinical findings.

▶ NURSING DIAGNOSIS: *Ineffective Breathing Pattern*

Related To
- Decreased lung expansion
- Decreased energy
- Fatigue
- Inflammatory process

Defining Characteristics
- Dyspnea
- Shortness of breath
- Cough
- Respiratory depth changes

Patient Outcomes
The patient will experience less discomfort due to changes in respiratory patterns.

Nursing Interventions	Rationales
Assist patient to assume position of comfort using pillows to support upper extremities.	An upright (Fowler's) position is generally more comfortable. Supporting the upper extremities avoids fatigue from strain on shoulders.

Nursing Interventions	Rationales
Avoid distention of bladder and bowel.	Distention of bladder and bowel diminishes lung expansion.
Allow adequate time for nursing care.	Rushing increases fatigue and can increase confusion.
Administer humidified oxygen therapy as prescribed. Use with caution in persons with underlying pulmonary disease.	Oxygen will prevent or alleviate hypoxia. One to 3 L of oxygen per minute is usually adequate for persons with obstructive lung disease.
Administer analgesics as prescribed.	Pain increases stress and tension, which can increase dyspnea.

▶ **NURSING DIAGNOSIS:** *High Risk for Fluid Volume Deficit*

Risk Factors
- Old age
- Physical immobility
- Increased metabolism related to inflammatory process
- Reluctance to drink due to functional incontinence

Patient Outcomes
The patient will maintain adequate fluid balance.

Nursing Interventions	Rationales
Assess for signs of dehydration: 1. thirst 2. decreased skin turgor 3. dry skin 4. dry mucus membranes 5. altered mental status 6. weakness 7. decreased pulse volume and increased rate **NOTE:** These signs may be absent or blunted in the elderly patient. Dry skin and decreased skin turgor may be due to aging.	Elderly patients can dehydrate rapidly, resulting in electrolyte imbalance.

Nursing Interventions	Rationales
Review laboratory data. Monitor fluid intake and output (I/O). Weigh daily.	
Question patient (if possible) regarding choices for fluids. Have fluids accessible. Instruct patient/family on need for adequate fluid intake. Assure patient that he or she will be assisted to bathroom as necessary.	Elderly persons may have limited range of motion, impaired vision, or other deficits that make it difficult to obtain fluids. Elderly persons often voluntarily restrict their fluid intake out of fear of incontinence.

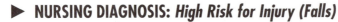 **NURSING DIAGNOSIS:** *High Risk for Injury (Falls)*

Risk Factors
- Altered internal regulatory function
- Fatigue
- Leukocytosis
- Altered mobility

Patient Outcomes
The patient will remain free of injury.

Nursing Interventions	Rationales
Assess patient for other risk factors for injury.	Preventive measures can be implemented.
Instruct patient to call for assistance when getting out of bed or out of the chair. Keep bed at lowest level.	The presence of infection diminishes strength, increasing the risk for falling during transfer procedures.
Allow to sit on the edge of the bed for a few seconds before coming to standing position. Have patient wear well-fitting shoes when walking.	Orthostatic hypotension increases the risk for falling. Improper foot wear reduces stability when walking.
Attend to patient's physical needs promptly.	A patient with unmet physical needs may not wait for assistance.

▶ NURSING DIAGNOSIS: *Altered Thought Processes*

Related To inflammatory process.

Defining Characteristics
- Disorientation
- Distractibility
- Memory deficits
- Hallucinations
- Delusions

Patient Outcomes
The patient will
- be treated effectively within the individual's abilities.
- be free of injuries resulting from altered thought processes.
- suffer minimal changes in mentation.

Nursing Interventions	Rationales
Assess for signs of cerebral irritation (see High Risk for Infection: Meningitis, page 129).	Altered thought processes may indicate complications of pneumonia, requiring medical treatment.
Assess extent of cognitive impairment (see Mini Mental Status Exam, Appendix D, page 349).	The degree of impairment dictates the type of interventions required. Additional safety measures may be needed.
Talk with family regarding previous history of cognitive impairment.	The patient may have a preexisting dementia such as Alzheimer's disease that is exacerbated by the infectious process.
Implement reality orientation procedures if disorientation is due to temporary acute illness. Provide supportive techniques if patient has diagnosis of dementia. (See Alzheimer's Disease, page 204.)	Reality orientation is ineffective for irreversible disorientation and may cause further agitation.

▶ NURSING DIAGNOSIS: *High Risk for Infection (Meningitis)*

Risk Factors
(See risk factors listed for pneumonia, page 338)
- History of influenza
- Pneumonia
- Gram negative meningitis becomes more common as people age

Patient Outcomes

The patient will
- receive interventions to prevent onset of meningitis.
- receive immediate treatment for signs and symptoms of meningitis.

Nursing Interventions	Rationales
Institute measures to prevent aspiration. Implement treatment for pneumonia.	The mouth frequently contains gram negative bacteria that can cause pneumonia when aspirated. Pneumonia is a risk factor for meningitis.
Monitor for signs and symptoms of meningitis in patients who are at risk: 1. severe headache 2. fever 3. malaise 4. diminishing consciousness 5. positive Kernig's sign (with patient in supine position, flex hip and knee and then straighten knee; note resistance or pain) 6. positive Brudzinski's sign (with patient in supine position, place hands behind patient's head and flex neck forward; note resistance or pain and flexion of hips and knees) NOTE: Remember that the elderly may not present obvious or typical manifestations.	Confusion may be ascribed to age or pneumonia, thus delaying treatment. Brudzinski's sign may be confused with cervical arthritis.
Prepare patient for prescribed diagnostic tests for meningitis: 1. lumbar puncture 2. blood cultures 3. computerized tomography (CT) scan or magnetic resonance imaging (MRI) studies	Early diagnosis and treatment is essential.

DISCHARGE PLANNING/CONTINUITY OF CARE

- Arrange for community services if necessary. Whether services are needed will depend on patient's preexisting health care needs, outcome of acute illness, and availability of a support system.
- Advise patient to obtain influenza vaccine every fall and pneumococcus vaccines after full recovery.
- Advise patient to avoid crowds during the flu season.

BIBLIOGRAPHY

Barzaga, R. A., & Cunha, B. A. (1992). Atypical pneumonia in the elderly. *Geriatric Focus on Infectious Diseases, 2*(3), 16, 12–14.

Bender, P. (1992). Deceptive distress in the elderly. *American Journal of Nursing, 92*(10), 29–33.

Falsey, A. R. (1991). Specific diagnosis of viral respiratory infections in the elderly. *Geriatric Focus on Infectious Diseases, 1*(3), 4–5, 11.

Fraser, D. (1993). Patient assessment—infection in the elderly. *Journal of Gerontological Nursing, 19*(7), 5–11.

Gluckman, S. J. (1992). Approach to the patient with pneumonia. In R. J. Duma (Ed.). *Recognition and management of nursing home infection.* Bethesda, MD: National Foundation for Infectious Diseases.

Keroack, M. A. (1991). The clinical challenge of pneumonia in the elderly. *Geriatric Focus on Infectious Diseases, 1*(3), 6–7, 10–11.

Mazanec, M. B. (1991). Importance of influenza and pneumococcal vaccines in the elderly. *Geriatric Focus on Infectious Diseases, 1*(3), 1–3.

$\mathcal{P}$ULMONARY TUBERCULOSIS

Pulmonary tuberculosis (TB) is a communicable disease spread by respiratory transmission through airborne droplet nuclei. The majority of individuals over 80 years of age who harbor the causative organism were infected as young adults. The organism resides in tubercles in a dormant stage for years. Reactivation of the disease may be triggered by chronic disease, poor nutrition, and long-term steroid use. Other persons at risk for acquiring tuberculosis are those who are as follows:
- human immunodeficiency virus (HIV) infected
- substance abusers
- prison inmates
- foreign-born persons from world areas with a high prevalence of TB
- ethnic groups known to have a high incidence of TB

Although pulmonary TB is the most common form of the disease, it is a systemic disease that can affect any body tissue or organ.

ETIOLOGIES
- Mycobacterium tuberculosis

CLINICAL MANIFESTATIONS
These typical signs of pulmonary TB may be absent in the elderly:
- fever
- night sweats
- cough
- increased sputum production
- weight loss
- hemoptysis
- chest pain

The elderly person may exhibit the following:
- difficulty breathing
- chronic cough

- general fatigue
- loss of appetite
- change in mental status

CLINICAL/DIAGNOSTIC FINDINGS

- Mantoux tuberculin skin test purified protein derivative (PPD): 5 tuberculin units (TU) in 0.1 mL solution intradermally: significant reaction (indurated area 10 mm or larger). Persons testing negative should be retested in 2 weeks to determine if booster effect has occurred. If the result on the second test is negative, repeat Mantoux test yearly.
- Chest x-ray: apical cavitary lesions (persons with HIV may have infiltrates in any lung zone or may have a normal chest x-ray).
- Sputum culture: acid-fast bacilli (AFB) found on three sputum specimens are collected on different days

NOTE: Persons with depressed immune systems may not exhibit a positive reaction to PPD even if active disease is present.

▶ NURSING DIAGNOSIS: *Altered Nutrition—Less Than Body Requirements*

Related To lack of appetite due to TB, coughing, and difficulty breathing.

Defining Characteristics

- Loss of 5% weight loss in 1 month, 7.5% loss over 3-month period or 10% loss over 6-month period
- Observed inadequate food intake

Patient Outcomes

The patient will
- maintain adequate nutritional status.
- attain usual/ideal body weight over a period of time.

Nursing Interventions	Rationales
Assess patient to determine reasons for altered nutrition: 1. cognitive impairment 2. presence of sensory/perceptual deficits (see page 225) 3. condition of oral cavity/dentures 4. dysphagia 5. ability to feed self 6. economic status 7. food likes/dislikes	There are many reasons for altered nutrition in the elderly. Interventions are based on the results of the assessment.

Nursing Interventions	Rationales
Offer several small meals a day with easy-to-chew, nourishing, high-calorie foods. Provide needed assistance. Use commercial thickeners for liquids if necessary.	It is important to conserve energy, avoiding fatigue during meals.
Monitor weight, weigh weekly.	Prompt detection of weight loss initiates prompt intervention.

▶ NURSING DIAGNOSIS: *Altered Protection*

Related To
- Inadequate nutrition
- Immune disorders
- Old age
- Drug therapies

Defining Characteristics
- Deficient immunity
- Disorientation
- Weakness, fatigue
- Chilling, perspiring
- Dyspnea
- Cough
- Anorexia

Patient Outcomes
The patient will be protected from situations that may increase the risk of acquiring complications.

Nursing Interventions	Rationales
Evaluate for risk of HIV infection.	Persons with HIV are at risk for contracting TB both from reactivation of a latent TB infection and from a new infection.
Protect from microorganisms transmitted through direct or indirect contact.	This will reduce the number of risk factors for infection. Patient is at risk for infection due to altered protection status.
Provide rest periods throughout the day. Encourage visitors to come during non–rest periods. Allow adequate time for nursing care to avoid rushing.	Avoid fatigue and dyspnea if possible.

Nursing Interventions	Rationales
Provide clock and calendar with large, easy-to-read numerals.	There is a high risk of disorientation during periods of isolation. Access to orienting information may prevent disorientation.
Determine cause of disorientation. If disorientation is reversible, apply reality orientation (RO) techniques.	Reality orientation techniques may prevent disorientation. If the disorientation is related to an underlying cognitive impairment such as Alzheimer's disease, the use of structured RO techniques will only serve to further frustrate patient and staff.
Maintain even environmental temperatures.	Avoid chilling and perspiring if possible.

▶ **NURSING DIAGNOSIS:** *Social Isolation*

Related To need for remaining in isolation in private room with door closed. (Duration of isolation is determined by clinical response and reduction in numbers of organisms on sputum culture. This is usually 2–3 weeks after chemotherapy is initiated.)

Defining Characteristics
- Absence of supportive others
- Uncommunicative
- Expresses feelings of aloneness imposed by others
- Feels "outcast" due to isolation

Patient Outcomes
The patient will be involved in activities of choice within the realm of the limits of isolation.

Nursing Interventions	Rationales
Provide patient with information regarding the need for isolation and when it may be discontinued. Encourage to practice acceptable personal hygiene to avoid	The patient needs full explanation for isolation within the realm of cognitive abilities to avoid feeling exiled. Occasional visits from staff may avoid formation of negative

Nursing Interventions	Rationales
transmitting organisms. Encourage staff to stop in room outside of times when care is rendered.	behaviors that may arise from feelings of loneliness.
Encourage short visits by family/significant others. Tell them that tuberculosis is not easily transmitted when proper precautions are implemented. Provide family with information about TB and instruct them on isolation procedures. Masks should be worn. Gloves are not necessary and gowns are not usually required unless contamination of clothing is likely.	Family/significant others may be reluctant to visit because of fear of exposure to disease.
Arrange for volunteer or activity aide to provide one-on-one diversional activities of patient's choice.	Group activities are not an option during the period of isolation. One-on-one activities with a person who can relate to the patient are an acceptable alternative.

▶ NURSING DIAGNOSIS: *Knowledge Deficit (Disease Process)*

Related To
- Lack of exposure to or misinterpretation of information
- Cognitive impairment
- Sensory deficits

Defining Characteristics
- Repeated questions about information that has been given many times
- Inappropriate behaviors concerning own welfare
- Relaying of misinformation to significant others

Patient Outcomes
The patient will
- verbalize understanding of disease process and treatment.
- identify relationship of clinical manifestations to the disease.
- initiate necessary life-style changes.

Nursing Interventions	Rationales
Evaluate level of knowledge about TB.	Instruction needs to start where the patient "is" at the time. Misinformation may need to be cleared up before new information is given.
Determine presence of barriers to learning (see Patient Teaching, Appendix C).	Persons with these problems may appear to comprehend but be hesitant to admit an inability to understand what is being taught. The presence of these problems may require alterations in teaching methods.
Establish priorities for learning and teach only what the patient needs to know, based on present knowledge base. Give positive reinforcement.	Persons relaying instructions may tend to "overteach," leaving the learner overwhelmed and frustrated. The patient needs encouragement and praise.

DISCHARGE PLANNING/CONTINUITY OF CARE

- Report to public health nurse in patient's county for follow-up investigation, evaluation, and treatment of contacts. (This should be done as soon as a diagnosis of TB is suspected.)
- Evaluate patient's ability to manage medication regime. Arrange for home health nurse or significant other to assume this responsibility if patient is unable to do so.
- Arrange for home health nurse to monitor for signs and symptoms of side effects of medications.
- Arrange for follow-up sputum testing to determine response to therapy. This should be done at least monthly until culture is negative.

Clinical Clip

- New cases of TB in the United States have increased 18%, reversing a 30-year downward trend. Multi-drug-resistant TB (MDRTB) strains of *M. tuberculosis* have become a concern. When organisms are resistant to the two most effective drugs, the course of treatment increases from 6 months to 18–24 months and the cure rate decreases from 100% to 60% or less. Administration of adjunctive therapy is recommended (see Table 15.2, page 140).

- Results of sputum cultures can now be obtained in 2 days instead of 3–4 weeks. Polymerase chain reaction (PCR) amplifies specific deoxyribonucleic acid (DNA) sequences for direct detection of the organism at the molecular level. *Mycobacterium* TB is detected with up to 99% sensitivity and 99% specificity.

Table 15.1 • Federal Regulations: Policy and Procedure for Occupational Exposure to Tuberculosis

The Occupational Safety and Health Act (OSHA) has developed legislation to enforce the recommendations of the Centers for Disease Control (CDC) for the control of TB in the workplace. These workplaces include the following:
- health care settings
- correctional institutions
- homeless shelters
- long-term care facilities for the elderly
- drug treatment centers

All OSHA requirements must be implemented at no cost to the employee.

The following is a summary of abatement methods required by OSHA for workplaces with occupational exposure:
1. The employer must provide and utilize a protocol for the early identification of individuals with TB.
2. The employer must provide medical surveillance, including
   - preplacement evaluation
   - administration and interpretation of TB Mantoux skin tests
   - periodic evaluations
     –initial baseline screening at time of employment for all employees
     –annually for all employees
     –every 6 months for employees with exposure as defined by CDC
3. The employer must provide evaluation and management of employees with any of the following:
   - positive skin test or with
   - skin test conversion on repeat testing
   - symptoms of TB

Table 15.1 • *continued*

- exposure to a patient with infectious TB for whom infection control precautions have not been taken
4. The employer must provide for placement of individuals with suspected or confirmed TB disease in an AFB isolation room. These rooms must be
    - maintained under negative pressure
    - appropriately exhausted
5. The employer must provide training and information to ensure employee knowledge.

Table 15.2 • Chemotherapy: Pulmonary Tuberculosis

Drug	Adverse Reactions	Monitor
Primary Therapy		
Isoniazid (INH)	Agranulocytosis, hemolytic anemia, peripheral neuropathy, hepatitis, hepatic enzyme elevation	Hepatic function studies, hematopoietic studies, signs of peripheral neuropathy
Rifampin	Hepatotoxicity; hemolytic anemia; affects action of oral contraceptives, quinidine, corticosteroids, digoxin, oral hypoglycemics	Hepatic function studies, hematopoietic studies, serum uric acid, symptoms of gout
Adjunctive Therapy		
Capreomycin sulfate	Neuromuscular blockade, ototoxicity, nephrotoxicity	Neuromuscular function, hearing evaluations, signs of ototoxicity, renal function, studies
Cycloserine	Seizures; possible suicidal tendencies; other psychiatric symptoms; side effects may be blocked by pyridoxine, ataractic agents, or anticonvulsants; impaired kidney and liver function	Psychiatric symptoms, hematology studies, renal and hepatic function studies
Ethambutol	Anaphylactoid reactions, elevated uric acid, diminished visual color, discrimination and visual acuity, impaired renal function	Visual acuity/color discrimination tests, serum uric acid, symptoms of gout, renal function studies

Table 15.2 • *continued*

Drug	Adverse Reactions	Monitor
Ethionamide	Hepatotoxicity, peripheral neuritis, anorexia, exfoliative dermatitis	Hepatic function studies, signs of peripheral neuropathy, skin rash
Pyrazinamide	Hepatotoxicity, hyperuricemia, arthralgia	Hepatic function studies, hematopoietic studies, serum uric acid, symptoms of gout and arthralgia.

BIBLIOGRAPHY

Boutotte, J. (1993a). T.B. The second time around. *Nursing 93, 23*(5), 42–49.

Boutotte, J. (1993b). Protecting yourself against T.B. *Nursing 93, 23*(10), 64.

Healthcare Pharmacy. (1992). Tuberculosis: New concern about an old disease. *LTC Nurse, 2*(12), 1, 3.

Tuberculosis: An old problem is new again. (1993). Molecular Biology Lab at Metpath. Corning Clinical Laboratory. M0039(3)1993. Teterboro, NJ.

U.S. Department of Health and Human Services. (1990a). Guidelines for preventing the transmission of tuberculosis in health-care settings, with special focus on HIV-related issues. *Morbidity & Mortality Weekly Report, 39*(RR–17).

U.S. Department of Health and Human Services. (1990b). Prevention and control of tuberculosis in facilities providing long-term care to the elderly. *Morbidity & Mortality Weekly Report, 39*(RR–10).

Wright, B. A. (1992). Tuberculosis surveillance program: A nursing home experience. *Geriatric Nursing, 13*(5), 257–261.

Gastrointestinal Conditions

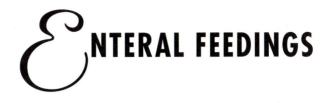
ENTERAL FEEDINGS

Administration of enteral tube feedings is a common procedure in hospitals, long-term care facilities, and the home. The feedings may be done on a temporary or permanent basis to maintain nutritional support.

ETIOLOGIES
- Neurological deficits resulting in dysphagia
- Radiation treatments to the head and neck
- Conditions involving severe catabolic stress

CLINICAL MANIFESTATIONS
Clinical manifestations are dependent on the need for the feeding:
- dysphagia
- inability to ingest oral intake to maintain adequate nutritional status

CLINICAL/DIAGNOSTIC FINDINGS
- Bedside evaluation by nurse or speech pathologist that indicates difficulty swallowing, choking, and drooling
- Video-recorded fluoroscopy to indicate dysphagia

▶ NURSING DIAGNOSIS: *Altered Nutrition—Less Than Body Requirements*

Related To feeding tube dislodgement.

Defining Characteristics
- Lack of nutritional intake
- Loss of weight

Patient Outcomes
The patient will
- have adequate nutritional intake.
- maintain or regain ideal weight.

Nursing Interventions	Rationales
Assist with or insert feeding tube immediately if it becomes dislodged.	Nutritional support is interrupted when enteral feeding ceases. Some feeding tube insertions require complex surgical procedures under general anesthesia. Others may be done at the bedside or as a minor procedure but require physician insertion, for example, percutaneous endoscopic gastrostomy (PEG) tubes. In some cases, the ostomy may heal within a few hours after tube removal, necessitating the reestablishment of the feeding access. In any of these situations, the patient may be without nourishment for several hours.
After tube is in place and after cleansing the area, use a transparent occlusive dressing to anchor feeding tube. If gauze dressing is used, tape tube securely to abdomen. [PEG or percutaneous endoscopic jejunostomy (PEJ) tubes do not need dressings after cleansing.] Investigate use of tube attachment devices and gastrostomy grips.	Adequate anchoring of tube will prevent dislodgement.
Monitor for coughing and vomiting.	Tubes are frequently dislodged because of coughing and vomiting. Appropriate interventions can be taken to prevent coughing and vomiting.
Monitor patient for agitation and pulling on tube. Assess for disorientation and confusion.	Confused patients may pull at the tube, causing dislodgement. Restraints should not be used. Use clothing to disguise and protect the tube. If the patient is not confused, the situation may need to be reevaluated to determine the patient's wishes.

Nursing Interventions	**Rationales**
Routinely check balloon on gastrostomy tubes: 1. Use universal precautions. 2. Remove fluid from balloon with Luer syringe. Compare volume of fluid with record of original amount instilled.	Routinely checking balloon volume prevents accidental removal of tube due to leakage of balloon.
Flush tubing regularly after determining placement: 1. Flush with 50 mL water before feedings are started and after they are completed. 2. Repeat flushing procedure every 4 h with continuous feedings. 3. Make sure diameter of tube is big enough to accommodate formula.	Prevent clogging of the tube.
Administer medications appropriately: 1. Never administer medications in formula. 2. Give in liquid form if available. 3. Crush pills finely and open capsules. Dissolve in warm water. (Ask pharmacist if this procedure is acceptable with specific medications.) 4. Dilute hypertonic medications with water prior to administration. 5. Flush tubing with water before and after administering medications. If feeding tube is clogged: 1. Use 50-mL piston syringe filled with 30 mL water and alternately push and pull on plunger (gently) to aspirate obstruction. NOTE: Many nurses report success with the use of colas, cranberry juice, and meat tenderizers for	Clogging may require the removal and reinsertion of the tube, placing the patient at risk for delays in nutritional intake.

Nursing Interventions	Rationales
declogging. The literature on this procedure is controversial. 2. If used, the solution must come into contact with the obstruction. Aspirate the feeding tube before instilling the solution. Avoid collapsing the tube. 3. Do not use meat tenderizer if the patient is allergic to papaya. 4. Instill 5–10 mL of solution with 30-mL syringe. Clamp tube, wait 15 min, and try to flush tube with water.	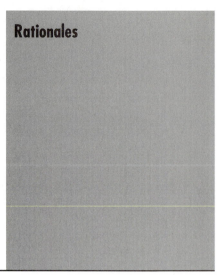

▶ **NURSING DIAGNOSIS:** *High Risk for Impaired Skin Integrity*

Risk Factors

Skin exposure to acidic and enzymatic fluids from stomach due to leakage around insertion site.

Patient Outcomes

The patient will remain free of impaired skin integrity.

Nursing Interventions	Rationales
Assess skin condition prior to tube insertion if possible.	Preexisting skin disease can be detected and treated. Sensitivity to adhesives or other topical treatments can be noted.
Observe daily for leakage and peristomial skin irritation.	Prompt remedial treatment can be initiated if tube is not positioned correctly: 1. Retention device should hold tube snugly against abdomen. 2. Fill balloon to correct volume.
Cleanse skin around stoma daily according to facility/agency policy:	Cleansing removes excretions and provides opportunity for skin

Nursing Interventions	Rationales
hydrogen peroxide (H_2O_2) followed by normal saline rinse, soap and water, or betadine. Apply gauze dressing or transparent occlusive dressing. The PEG and PEJ sites require no dressing after cleansing. If leakage is present, apply skin barrier.	inspection. Skin barrier protects skin from drainage.
Position patient on right side during and for 1–2 h after feeding.	The position of the stomach prevents leakage.
Remove feeding tube and discontinue gastric feedings if skin integrity becomes impaired. (Parenteral nutrition will need to be implemented for this period). Insert smaller, rubber, silicone catheter.	This promotes shrinkage of the ostomy around the smaller device. Suction or gravity drainage is attached to curb the gastric secretions. After the size is decreased, progressively larger tubes are inserted until a tight closure is attained.

▶ **NURSING DIAGNOSIS:** *High Risk for Aspiration*

Risk Factors
- Tube feeding
- Increased gastric residual
- Decreased gastric motility
- Delayed gastric emptying
- Reduced level of consciousness
- Depressed cough and gag reflex

Patient Outcomes
The patient will remain free of aspiration.

Nursing Interventions	Rationales
Check tube placement before each feeding and at least once a day for continuous feedings. 1. Place stethoscope over epigastric area and inject 5 mL of air into	Checking tube placement decreases risk of aspiration.

Nursing Interventions	**Rationales**
tubing. A whooshing sound should indicate correct placement. 2. Aspirate gastric contents. 3. Check aspirated fluids for pH. Acidic pH (1.0–4.0) should be an indication of stomach placement. Alkaline pH may indicate small bowel or lung placement.	
When initiating tube feedings, administer formula slowly for first 24 h at a rate of 25–30 mL/h and use one-half concentration. If there are no complications, gradually increase rate. After desired rate is reached, gradually increase concentration to full strength. Use pump on continuous feedings to control rate.	Feeding too fast can cause vomiting, resulting in aspiration.
Check gastric residual before each intermittent feeding and once q4h for continuous feedings. Aspirate gastric contents, measure, and return to patient's stomach. If more than 100 mL was removed, wait for $\frac{1}{2}$–1 h and recheck. If there is still more than 100 mL, notify physician.	A large amount of residual increases risk of aspiration.
Avoid bolus feedings into the stomach.	Bolus feedings into the stomach may cause abdominal distention and increase the risk of aspiration. NOTE: The dumping syndrome can occur if bolus feedings are used for feedings into the duodenum or jejunum.
Elevate head of bed 30° during continuous feedings. Maintain this position for 1 h after intermittent feedings.	Gastroesophageal reflux is prevented.
Monitor for signs and symptoms of pneumonia: infiltrates in lung fields on x-ray, cough, dyspnea, fever, chest pain, and sputum production.	The pneumonia may be a result of aspiration. The situation needs to be evaluated to prevent recurrence.

▶ NURSING DIAGNOSIS: *Diarrhea*

Related To incompatibility of feeding formula.

Defining Characteristics
* Abdominal pain
* Cramping and urgency
* Increased frequency of stools
* Increased frequency of bowel sounds
* Loose, liquid stools

Patient Outcomes
The patient will
* be free of discomfort related to diarrhea.
* resume usual bowel elimination habits.

Nursing Interventions	Rationales
When initiating tube feedings, administer formula slowly for first 24 h at a rate of 25–30 mL/h and use one-half concentration.	A too rapid rate and full concentration can cause diarrhea.
Evaluate medication regime.	Diarrhea in persons receiving tube feedings frequently occurs with concurrent antibiotic use.
Administer continuous or intermittent feedings rather than bolus feedings.	Patients receiving continuous feedings experience fewer episodes of diarrhea than those receiving bolus doses.
Check for lactose intolerance.	Lactose intolerance can cause diarrhea.
Assist patient to use commode or toilet for defecation.	Gravity promotes bowel emptying and diminishes oozing stool.

▶ NURSING DIAGNOSIS: *Diversional Activity Deficit*

Related To tube feedings.

Defining Characteristics
* Complaints of boredom
* Desire to be more active and involved

Patient Outcomes

The patient will
- participate in activities of choice.
- feel relieved of boredom.

Nursing Interventions	Rationales
Change from continuous or intermittent feeding to cyclic feeding.	Cyclic feedings can be administered over a 12–16-h period during the evening and night. The patient is not encumbered by feeding equipment during the day and will have more freedom to participate in activities.
Monitor for tolerance as the same amount of formula will be administered over a shorter period of time.	The same amount of formula will be administered over a shorter period of time if feedings are switched from continuous to cyclic.
If cyclic feedings are not an alternative, make arrangements for the patient to be out of the room for a few hours each day, by moving the bed or utilizing a lounge chair.	A change of scene can provide sensory stimulation.
Ask patient about previous hobbies and pastimes.	If the patient enjoys solitary activities, appropriate items can be provided: books, needlework, listening to music, watching television, or puzzles.

DISCHARGE PLANNING/CONTINUITY OF CARE

If patient is going home:
- Make sure that patient/family are able to administer feedings and provide peristomial care and can monitor for complications.
- Provide family with information for obtaining supplies and determine source of payment.
- Assess for home equipment needs: hospital bed, commode, or shower chair.
- Arrange for home health nurse to visit periodically to evaluate situation.

If patient is going to long-term care facility:

- Provide facility with complete information regarding type of feeding tube, route of feeding, type of formula, and complications that have occurred.

Clinical Clip

Gastrostomy tubes can migrate inward (causing nausea, vomiting, and abdominal distention) or outward (causing pain, redness, swelling, and abdominal drainage). Check length of tube, stop feedings, and contact physician.

BIBLIOGRAPHY

Bockus, S. (1993). When your patient needs tube feedings. *Nursing 93, 23*(7), 3434–3442.

Bodner, B., & Fraher, J. (1989). Tube feeding enterostomies: Indications, techniques, and management strategies. *Progressions, 1*(2), 54, 56, 58–61.

Fuller, N. A., & Lawrence, K. G. (1992). How to stabilize a percutaneous tube. *Nursing 92, 22*(7), 52–54.

Galindo-Ciocon, D. J. (1993). Tube feeding: Complications among the elderly. *Journal of Gerontological Nursing, 19*(6), 17–22.

Murray, M. (1993). Principles of caring for residents with feeding tubes. *Nursing Homes, 42*(9), 37–39.

Parrington, D. J., & Rousseau, P. (1993). Enteral feeding of nursing home residents. *Nursing Home Medicine, 1*(3), 14, 17–19, 22–23.

Raymond, J. L. (1992). Updated guidelines for tube feeding. *Nursing Homes, 41*(6), 33–34.

Webber-Jones, J., et al. (1992). Declogging a feeding tube. *Nursing 92, 22*(4), 63–64.

ℱECAL DIVERSIONS

Because of increased life expectancy, more elderly people are undergoing stomal surgery. After 5 or 6 days in the hospital, the individual returns home or to a long-term care facility. Ostomy surgery at any age can be devastating and is no less so for the elderly patient. The changes associated with aging, such as sensory impairments, skin changes, and diminishing fine motor coordination, increase the challenges faced by the patient and the caregiver. Colostomies are the most common type of ostomy performed in geriatric patients.

ETIOLOGIES
- Colostomy (sigmoid and descending, usually in conjunction with partial colectomy)
  - cancer of the rectum or sigmoid colon
  - chronic diverticulitis
- Colostomy (transverse, often temporary)
  - perforating sigmoid diverticulitis
  - recto-vaginal fistula
  - penetrating trauma
  - obstructing, inoperable tumor in colon, rectum, or pelvis
- Colostomy (ascending, same as transverse)

CLINICAL MANIFESTATIONS
Dependent on need for surgery

CLINICAL/DIAGNOSTIC FINDINGS
- Examination of stool for occult blood: positive for gastrointestinal benign or malignant tumors, ulcerations, inflammation
- Barium enema study (lower gastrointestinal series): identifies tumors and polyps
- Colonoscopy/sigmoidoscopy: identifies lesions, tumors, inflammation, ulceration

▶ **NURSING DIAGNOSIS:** *High Risk for Impaired Skin Integrity*

Risk Factors
- Skin changes resulting from aging
- Drainage/fecal material from stoma
- Unsuitable appliance

Patient Outcomes
The patient will be free of skin impairment.

Nursing Interventions	Rationales
NOTE: Teach patient each step of the procedure. Supervise performance and determine when the patient is ready to assume this responsibility. (See Appendix C, Patient Teaching, page 345.) Change pouching system as necessary. Pouching systems are changed from 2 to 14 days depending on the type of system. Change immediately if system is leaking. Always empty pouch when it is one-third to one-half full.	Changing the system as infrequently as possible minimizes skin breakdown around the stoma. Leakage and overflow of contents increases the risk of skin breakdown.
Wipe stoma and peristomial area gently with facial tissue. Then wash and dry peristomial skin. Inspect skin and stoma.	Cleanliness minimizes risk of skin breakdown.
Apply pouch. Before applying adhesive-backed pouch with separate skin barrier, measure stoma and trace size opening from measuring guide onto the back of the barrier's adhesive side. Cut out opening, making it $\frac{1}{8}$ in. larger than tracing. If pouch has precut openings, select one that is $\frac{1}{8}$ in. larger than stoma. Stoma paste may be applied to the back of the skin barrier for patients with ileostomies or ascending colostomies.	Pouch openings that are too big allow leakage. An opening that is constrictive can injure the stoma or skin without the patient's awareness because there are no pain receptors in the stoma.

Nursing Interventions	Rationales
NOTE: Specific application depends on the type and brand of product that is selected.	

▶ NURSING DIAGNOSIS: *Bowel Incontinence*

Related To irregular bowel function due to colostomy.

Defining Characteristics
Unpredictability of bowel movements

Patient Outcomes
The patient will establish a predictable bowel elimination pattern.

Nursing Interventions	Rationales
Prepare patient for colostomy irrigation. The procedure may be done in bed or in the bathroom.	Bowel function regularity of a descending or sigmoid colostomy can be established by irrigation because solid bowel contents are stored there. For this reason, irrigation is not effective for ascending colostomies or ileostomies. The procedure can be initiated as soon as bowel function returns after surgery.
Advise patient to avoid 1. gas-forming foods such as beans and vegetables from the cabbage group. 2. foods with seeds or shells such as nuts and corn because they can cause a mechanical obstruction. Advise drinking plenty of fluids.	Diet and fluid intake also is a factor in bowel function. Irrigation alone cannot regulate the bowel.
Evaluate medication regime.	Patient may be taking laxatives which are not necessary with an ascending colostomy. If constipation is a problem with a descending or sigmoid colostomy, prune

Nursing Interventions	Rationales
	juice or psyllium hydrophilic mucilloid should be effective. For patients with ascending colostomies, enteric-coated medications may not be completely absorbed before being expelled through stoma. A liquid form may need to be substituted.
Advise regular exercise appropriate to patient's physical condition and abilities.	Exercise promotes bowel regularity.

▶ **NURSING DIAGNOSIS:** *Knowledge Deficit (Colostomy Care)*

Related To surgery and resulting colostomy.

Defining Characteristics
- Verbalization of lack of knowledge concerning colostomy
- Request for information
- Verbalization of willingness to care for colostomy

Patient Outcomes
The patient will
- participate in learning process.
- verbalize understanding of colostomy.
- correctly perform daily colostomy care.

Nursing Interventions	Rationales
Assess readiness to learn. Observe for indications of denial and avoidance.	Learning will not be successful until the patient is ready to accept the colostomy and the information that is presented.
Assess ability to learn (see Patient Teaching, Appendix C, page 345).	Elderly people require direct, nonglare lighting and bold print for visual learning. A magnifying glass may be needed. Utilize communication skills for hearing impairments (see Hearing Impairment, page 278). Present

Nursing Interventions	Rationales
	information in private, quiet place, free of environmental noise. If cognitive and/or self-care deficits are present, include a family member in the teaching sessions.
Attend to physical needs prior to learning sessions: 1. bladder elimination 2. hunger/thirst 3. pain 4. fatigue	Physical needs override the need to learn.
Present information in small segments. Evaluate learning before proceeding to next segment. Reinforce information and provide encouragement.	There is a limit to the amount of information that can be absorbed at one time.

▶ NURSING DIAGNOSIS: *Body Image Disturbance*

Related To surgery and changes in bowel function.

Defining Characteristics
- Verbalization of fears of rejection or reaction of others
- Verbalization of negative feelings about body
- Not looking at surgical area during care
- Unwillingness to participate in care of stoma

Patient Outcomes
The patient will
- verbalize acceptance of self and of changes in body
- assume responsibility for stoma care (if mentally and physically capable)

Nursing Interventions	Rationales
Instruct caregivers (professional or family/significant others) to be aware of personal feelings about the surgery that may be revealed in their body language.	Feelings of repulsion or disgust can be readily evident in facial expressions and other nonverbal cues. This reinforces the patient's negative perceptions.

Nursing Interventions	Rationales
Allow patient to ventilate feelings and concerns.	Empathy from caregivers may lead to acceptance by the patient. Listening may reveal misconceptions that need to be clarified.
Discuss adaptations in life-style that will allow the patient to continue with high-priority activities.	The patient may be more accepting of the body changes if previous life-style can be resumed.
Avoid thrusting the patient into caring for the stoma before he or she is ready.	It takes time to overcome initial feelings of shock and denial that accompany major body changes.
Select stoma equipment that is simple to use, readily available, and cost-effective. Use as few items as possible.	Acceptance will not occur if the patient is overwhelmed with the care and equipment.
Obtain patient's permission to arrange a visit from another person with a colostomy who is about the same age. Contact the local chapter of the United Ostomy Association.	Seeing another person of the same generation with an ostomy who is active, accepting, and contented can boost the morale of the patient. The visitor can answer questions concerning resuming of social activities.
Provide information and support pertaining to sexuality and sexual activity if patient is sexually active.	Caregivers may wrongly assume that elderly patients do not have concerns about sexuality. Sexuality is a life-long characteristic and may or may not include coitus. Elderly patients may be reluctant to verbalize concerns.

DISCHARGE PLANNING/CONTINUITY OF CARE

If patient is going home:
- Arrange for home health nurse to evaluate progress in self-care and to assess need for additional teaching.
- Provide information for purchasing of stoma supplies and equipment. Determine source of payment for supplies.
- Arrange for other services as required by patient's mental and physical status: home delivered meals, home health aide, or homemaker.

If patient is transferring to long-term care facility, provide information on
- status of patient teaching.
- progress toward acceptance of ostomy.

- procedure for ostomy care and irrigation.
- type of supplies being used.

BIBLIOGRAPHY

Kuhn, J. K., & Flaherty, M. J. M. (1990). Helping ostomy patients back to independence. *Journal of Gerontological Nursing, 16*(6), 27–30.

Loeb, S. (Ed.). (1992). Gastrointestinal care. *Nursing procedures.* Springhouse, PA: Springhouse Corporation.

Long, L. (1991). Ileostomy care. *Nursing 91, 22*(10), 73–75.

Urological Tract Conditions

URINARY INCONTINENCE

Urinary incontinence is not a disease, nor is it a normal, expected aging change. However, urinary incontinence is a frequent problem for older adults because of physiological changes related to aging: These include diminished estrogen levels in females and enlarged prostate in males. Disease processes causing cognitive or mobility impairment and medications can increase the risk of incontinence. There are six major types of urinary incontinence: stress, reflex, urge, functional, total, and overflow. More than one type may be present in an individual at the same time.

ETIOLOGIES
- Transient causes
  - medication
  - acute illness
  - recent removal of indwelling catheter
  - recent surgery of genitourinary tract
  - local irritation
- Complex causes
  - overactive detrusor
  - underactive detrusor
  - urethral instability

CLINICAL MANIFESTATIONS
Inability to control discharge of urine from bladder at appropriate time and in appropriate place

CLINICAL/DIAGNOSTIC FINDINGS
- Physical examination to rule out
  - tumors
  - genital abnormalities
  - atrophy
  - pelvic prolapse
- Assessment and history (see Table 18.1, page 175)

- Additional tests that may be performed:
  - estimation of postvoid residual (PVR) volume: >200 mL considered inadequate emptying
  - provocative stress testing: instant urine leakage indicating stress incontinence; if leakage delayed or persists after cough, suspect detrusor overactivity
  - urinalysis: if positive for bacteria and/or white blood cells, request urine culture to rule out infection as cause of incontinence
  - urodynamic testing: uroflowmetry (abnormal voiding patterns), cystometry (voluntary and involuntary detrusor contractions)
  - endoscopy imaging: bladder lesions, foreign bodies, urethral diverticula, fistula, strictures
  - cytology: malignancy

▶ NURSING DIAGNOSIS: *Functional Incontinence*

Related To
- Impaired mobility, loss of manual dexterity required for manipulation of clothing during toileting
- Impaired vision/inability to find toilet
- Unfamiliar environment
- Unusually large output related to diuretics, diabetes, or increased intake of fluids
- Disorientation
- Loss of motivation
- Depression, anger, frustration, or perceived rewards associated with incontinence

Defining Characteristics
- Involuntary passage of urine is unpredictable and complete.
- Body language or behavioral changes may be noted in persons who are cognitively impaired. They are often aware of the need to void but cannot act on the need without assistance.
- Frustration and anger may be noted in persons who are physically impaired.

Patient Outcomes
The patient will remain dry.

Nursing Interventions	Rationales
Complete an assessment (See Table 18.1, page 175) to determine cause of functional incontinence.	Management of functional incontinence is dependent on the cause.

Nursing Interventions	Rationales
Arrange environment to facilitate toileting if this is the cause. Placement of a commode or use of signs showing direction to bathroom may help.	Functional incontinence may be a result of inability to reach the bathroom due to environmental causes.
Assess for mobility training.	If the patient has impaired physical mobility, increasing mobility skills may prevent the incontinence.
Implement habit-training program (see Reflex Incontinence), scheduled toileting, or prompted voiding for patients whose functional incontinence is a result of cognitive impairment: 1. Scheduled toileting: Take the patient to the bathroom every 2 h during waking hours. 2. Prompted voiding: Take the patient to the bathroom at regularly scheduled intervals and give social reinforcement for appropriate toileting behavior.	The goal is to have the patient remain dry. Cognitively impaired patients are dependent on staff to assist them to the bathroom at the scheduled times. They are not able to participate in retraining or other programs.
Consider use of external catheter devices if toileting programs are not effective. These are available for women as well as men but may not be practical in a woman who is cognitively impaired.	The goal of remaining dry can be attained even though other methods are unsuccessful.

▶ **NURSING DIAGNOSIS:** *Stress Incontinence*

Related To
- Weakness of the urethral sphincter or weakened pelvic floor musculature causing abdominal pressure to exceed urethral resistance
- Females: urethral or vaginal prolapse, cystocele, rectocele, atrophic vaginitis, obesity, chronic overdistention, and multiple pregnancies are contributing factors
- Males: damage to the proximal urethra during transurethral prostatectomy

Defining Characteristics
- Involuntary passage of urine associated with coughing, laughing, straining, or other physical activity that increases abdominal pressure
- Dribbling, frequency, urgency

Patient Outcomes
The patient will
- experience fewer episodes of incontinence.
- demonstrate ability to perform Kegel exercises.
- verbalize knowledge of personal hygiene techniques.
- verbalize understanding of cause of incontinence.

Nursing Interventions	Rationales
Teach Kegel exercises if patient has adequate cognitive function: 1. Sit on toilet with knees apart and feet flat on floor. 2. Tighten the ring of muscle around the anus as though trying to hold back a bowel movement. Do this without tensing the muscles of the legs, buttocks, or abdomen.	The patient can identify the back part of the pelvic floor.
Stop the flow of urine while voiding, hold for a few seconds, and then restart the flow.	The patient learns to identify the front part of the pelvic floor.
This exercise can be done any time, while sitting or standing: 1. Slowly tighten the muscles from front to back while counting to 4. 2. Then release muscles. 3. Do not tighten abdominal, thigh, or buttock muscles or cross the legs. Women can check the effectiveness by placing one finger inside the vagina and contracting the muscles. Improved urine control is the only way that men can check for success.	The pelvic floor muscles and the squeezing action of the urethra are strengthened.
With every urination: start and stop the stream five times.	The pelvic floor musculature and squeezing action are strengthened. The urethra is eventually able to overcome the abdominal pressure.

Nursing Interventions	Rationales
Discuss the reasons for the exercises and the complications of incontinence.	Knowledge facilitates compliance with exercise regime.
Encourage loss of excess weight. Arrange for consultation with dietitian if possible for nutrition education.	Weight loss decreases abdominal pressure.
Use incontinence briefs during waking hours until continence is stable.	The briefs keep urine away from the skin. The patient is able to socialize without fear of embarrassment.
Instruct in perineal cleansing and to wipe from front to back after toileting.	Cleanliness prevents odor and skin irritation. Wiping from front to back minimizes introduction of bacteria to urethral area, reducing risk of infection.
Instruct to void as soon as urge is felt.	Overdistention of bladder increases pressure on urethra, increasing the possibility of incontinence.
Consult with physician on administration of oral estrogen tablets.	The urethra and vagina are sensitive to decreased hormone production. Symptoms may be noted several years after menopause is completed and are a major cause of stress incontinence. For aesthetic reasons, increased compliance has been noted with oral estrogen as opposed to estrogen creams that need to be vaginally inserted.
Consult with physician regarding possibility of surgical intervention if Kegel exercises are not effective and patient is candidate for surgery. Surgical techniques elevate or suspend the urethra and provide support during activities that create stress or straining.	Persistent incontinence can cause severe skin impairment, predispose to urinary tract infections, and generate social isolation and diminished self-esteem.

► NURSING DIAGNOSIS: *Reflex Incontinence*

Related To
- Central nervous system or spinal cord disease or injury
- Impaired transmission of signals from reflex arc to cerebral cortex

Defining Characteristics
- Involuntary passage of urine related to uninhibited bladder contractions and spasms, often establishing a predictable pattern
- Diminished or absent awareness of bladder fullness and urge to void

Patient Outcomes
The patient will
- experience freedom from incontinence.
- verbalize understanding of cause of incontinence.
- comply with regime based on habit-training program.
- verbalize knowledge of personal hygiene techniques.

Nursing Interventions	Rationales
Record times of incontinence for several days.	Analysis of the incontinent record may reveal a predictable pattern of voiding. A schedule can then be established.
Establish a habit-training program based on the pattern of voiding. Instruct caregivers to toilet patient on a schedule based on the incontinent record.	The patient will remain dry by emptying the bladder just prior to the predicted time of incontinence.
Consult with physician regarding administration of anticholinergic medication.	Medication relaxes bladder, preventing uninhibited contractions, thereby avoiding incontinence.

► NURSING DIAGNOSIS: *Urge Incontinence*

Related To
- Bladder irritation from infections, tumors, stones, ingestion of certain foods, beverages
- Enlarged prostate
- Atrophic vaginitis
- Decreased bladder capacity as a consequence of an indwelling catheter or abdominal surgery
- Increased urine concentration
- Overdistention of bladder

Defining Characteristics
- Involuntary passage of urine occurring immediately after sensation of bladder fullness perceived
- Voiding more frequently than every 2 h
- Voiding in small amounts (<100 mL) or in large amounts (>500 mL)
- Frequency, nocturia

Patient Outcomes
The patient will
- experience fewer incontinent episodes.
- verbalize understanding of cause of incontinence.
- comply with regime based on cause of incontinence.
- verbalize knowledge of personal hygiene techniques.

Nursing Interventions	Rationales
Rule out local genitourinary conditions and central nervous system (CNS) disorders.	Management is based on cause of incontinence.
Instruct to avoid coffee, tea, cola, and alcohol.	Caffeine-containing beverages and alcohol may cause irritation to the bladder and often have a diuretic effect.
Consult with physician regarding administration of estrogen for female patient.	Atrophic vaginitis/urethritis will respond to this treatment (see Stress Incontinence, page 167).
Implement bladder-retraining program if patient is cognitively unimpaired and has adequate physical mobility.	Patient must be able to understand and cooperate with the program. Physical mobility may not be a major consideration if a caregiver is available throughout the day to assist the patient to the bathroom as scheduled.
Toilet patient upon awakening, at bedtime, q2h during the day, and q4h during the night. Maintain voiding record and document times and amounts of voiding and whether patient was continent or incontinent. Maintain fluid intake records.	A pattern can be established based on ability to remain continent between voiding times.

Nursing Interventions	Rationales
Encourage to delay voiding until scheduled time. Instruct patient on techniques for bladder emptying: bending forward, exerting gentle suprapubic pressure, or double voiding.	The feeling of urgency may be delayed. Emptying the bladder completely ensures less feeling of urgency and increases probability for success in remaining continent.
Increase times gradually between voidings if patient has been able to remain continent until established voiding times.	Attempt to increase bladder capacity before signs of urgency are present.
Decrease times between voidings if patient is incontinent or is unable to wait until scheduled voiding times.	Avoid incontinence and further evaluate situation to determine bladder capacity.
Do PVR if patient has consistent inability to follow established voiding times.	If the bladder is not being emptied with each void, the patient will experience urgency much sooner. A large PVR may indicate a need for further investigation of the problem.
Continue with program by attempting to increase times between voidings. If patient is unable to tolerate the delayed voiding, maintain the initial schedule.	The goal is to remain continent. Patient may have to continue with toileting q2h to attain this goal.
Consult with physician regarding medication if patient continues to have urgency and incontinence: propantheline, flavoxate, dicyclomine, imipramine, oxybutynin, and hyoscyamine sulfate.	The first three medications work by decreasing bladder contractions. Imipramine decreases bladder contractions and tightens the sphincter muscle. The last two medications increase bladder capacity.

▶ **NURSING DIAGNOSIS:** *Total Incontinence*

Related To lack of awareness of bladder filling or emptying.

NOTE: This classification is used when all other types of incontinence have been ruled out.

Defining Characteristics
- Unpredictable, involuntary, continuous loss of urine
- Absence of distention or uninhibited bladder contractions
- Nocturia

Patient Outcomes
The patient will experience freedom from impaired skin integrity as a result of the incontinence.

Nursing Interventions	Rationales
Utilize absorbent incontinent pads or briefs. When selecting a product, consider absorbency, bulk, comfort, availability, cost, ease of changing, and disposability.	Total incontinence is not generally amenable to behavior management programs. The goal is to prevent skin breakdown from the urine. Incontinent pads and briefs have a wicking action that draws the urine away from the skin, decreasing the risk of skin breakdown.
Implement program of skin cleanliness: 1. Check pads/briefs q2h for wetness. 2. Cleanse buttocks, groin, and perineal area thoroughly after each incontinent episode with a wash made for this purpose.	Cleanliness avoids skin breakdown. Most soaps are alkaline and tend to irritate the skin. It is often difficult to remove all soap residue. Washes that do not require rinsing are more effective.
Apply a moisture barrier after cleaning.	Ointments are often difficult to remove. Talcum powder has a tendency to "bead" when mixed with moisture and causes excoriation of the skin. Corn starch encourages bacterial growth. Moisture barriers protect the skin without the hazards of ointments or powders.
Inspect skin for evidence of skin breakdown with each incontinent episode. Check legs frequently for skin irritation, especially if patient is ambulatory.	Incontinence increases the risk of impaired skin integrity. Leakage from the briefs may occur, trickling down the leg, causing skin irritation.

▶ NURSING DIAGNOSIS: *Overflow Incontinence*

Related To retention due to
- obstruction from enlarged prostate, stricture, or cystocele, fecal impaction
- acontractile bladder due to diabetes or spinal cord injury

Defining Characteristics
- Chronic inability to void with bladder distention
- Small frequent voidings or dribbling

Patient Outcomes
The patient will
- experience freedom from dribbling and incontinence.
- experience complete bladder emptying at regular intervals.

Nursing Interventions	Rationales
Rule out the presence of obstruction.	Removing the obstruction should allow for the free passage of urine through the urethra.
Implement program of intermittent catheterization q3–4h during the day and as necessary at night if obstruction has been ruled out. Clean intermittent catheterization (CIC) is appropriate for patients at home. Sterile procedure is recommended for institutional settings.	Clean intermittent catheterization reduces the incidence of urinary tract infections, reflux, renal and bladder stones, and hydro-ureteronephrosis. The risk of infection is much less for the patient at home, making clean technique a practical and safe procedure.
Teach patient procedure if possible.	Advocates of CIC believe that age is not a factor in self-catheterization if manual dexterity is present. Increased independence is possible if self-catheterization is possible. NOTE: Indwelling catheters are the treatment of choice only if a behavioral program to improve bladder function has been attempted and failed, CIC is not practical, or the use of absorbent products is inappropriate (see Table 18.2, page 176).

DISCHARGE PLANNING/CONTINUITY OF CARE

- Provide written instructions if patient is doing Kegel exercises.
- Inform patient where catheterization supplies may be purchased if patient will be performing self-CIC.
- Provide instructions for catheter care if patient has indwelling catheter.
- Inform patient/family where incontinent briefs/pads may be purchased.
- Instruct patient to maintain adequate fluid intake and to report signs of urinary tract infection to physician.

Table 18.1 • Assessment for Bladder Management

Patient _____ Admission No._____ Date _____
Diagnoses _____ Birthdate _____

Bladder function
History of infection or other urinary problem _____

Previous treatment and effects _____

Other lower urinary tract symptoms _____

Duration of incontinence_____
Alterations in bowel habits _____
Alterations in sexual habits _____
Observe voiding for hesitancy, straining, force of stream, interruption in
stream_____

Medications affecting bladder function/continence

_____

Mental status
Short-term memory_____Orientation _____
Able to express self _____ Able to follow directions _____
Reaction to incontinence _____
Hydration baseline
Daily average fluid intake: days _____ evenings _____ nights _____
Mobility/self-care skills
Ambulatory/self_____Cane _____Walker _____

Requires Assist of 1–2_____Weight Bearing_____

Propels self with cane _____Transfers self_____
Requires assistance _____
Can manage clothing _____
Cleans self after toileting _____
Washes hands _____

Table 18.1 • *continued*

To be completed after 2-week assessment period

Frequency of voiding _____average amt. _____

Is patient aware of need to void? _____Urgency? _____

Dribbling? _____Incontinence preceded by laughing, sneezing? _____

Evaluation for management of program

Plan_____

Rationale _____

Nurse _____

Table 18.2 • Guidelines for Use and Care of Indwelling Catheters

Clinical conditions indicating the need for an indwelling catheter:

1. urinary retention with persistent overflow incontinence
2. symptomatic infections and/or renal dysfunction
3. skin wounds or pressure ulcers that are contaminated by urine
4. terminally ill or severely impaired patients for whom changes of clothing and linen are uncomfortable or disruptive

Indwelling Catheter Care

1. Catheterization procedures should be carried out only by persons with knowledge of the procedure and sterile technique.
2. Wash hands thoroughly before and after any manipulation of the catheter site or apparatus.
3. Use universal precautions when there is the possibility of contact with urine.
4. Use as small a catheter as possible with as small a balloon as possible to minimize uretheral trauma. A No. 16 catheter with 5-mL balloon is usually adequate. Leaking around the catheter does not justify the use of a larger catheter.
5. Secure the catheter after insertion to prevent movement and urethral traction.
6. Maintain a sterile, closed drainage system. Irrigation or changing to a leg bag are the only exceptions.
7. Keep drainage bag below the level of the bladder.
8. Disinfect catheter/tubing junction before disconnecting.
9. Date tubing and drainage bag and change regularly.
10. Empty drainage bag at least once q8h. Use a separate collecting container for each patient. The spigot should not touch the container.

BIBLIOGRAPHY

Faller, N. (1992). Clean intermittent catheterization. *Ostomy/Wound Management, 38*(7), 29, 30, 34–37.

Haight, B. K., & Wells, T. J. (1992). Urinary incontinence: Two viewpoints. *Journal of Gerontological Nursing, 18*(6), 41–46.

Needham, J. (1993). *Gerontological nursing, a restorative approach.* Albany, NY: Delmar.

Ouslander, J. D., Ditzler, J. L., & Brandeis, G. (1993). Managing urinary incontinence. *Nursing Homes, 42*(2), 21–27.

U.S. Department of Health and Human Services. Agency for Health Care Policy and Research. (1992). *Urinary incontinence in adults. Clinical practice guidelines.* U.S. Department of Health and Human Services. Rockville, MD.

Warkentine, R. (1992). Implementation of a urinary continence program. *Journal of Gerontological Nursing, 18*(1), 31–36.

$\mathcal{U}$RINARY TRACT INFECTION

$\mathbf{U}$rinary tract infections are a common cause of acute illness in the elderly. They are more common in women than in men due to the shorter urethra and proximity to the vaginal and rectal orifices.

ETIOLOGIES
- *Escherichia coli*
- *Klebsiella pneumoniae*
- *Proteus mirabilis*
- *Enterococcus*
- *Streptococcus*

CLINICAL MANIFESTATIONS
- Typical symptoms
  - fever
  - dysuria
  - urgency, frequency of urination
  - suprapubic tenderness
- Common symptoms in the elderly
  - incontinence
  - onset or increase in confusion
  - decrease in activity
  - decrease in appetite
  - unexplained tachycardia or tachypnea
  - unexplained falls

CLINICAL/DIAGNOSTIC FINDINGS
Laboratory findings:
- culture positive for bacteria
- bacterial counts >10^5 colonies/mL urine
- pyuria ≥10 white blood cells (WBC)/mL^3 or ≥3 WBC/high-power field of unspun urine

The diagnosis must also be supported by the presence of clinical criteria as described under Clinical Manifestations.

▶ NURSING DIAGNOSIS: *Altered Urinary Elimination*

Related To bacteriuria.

Defining Characteristics
- Incontinence
- Decrease in activity
- Decrease in appetite

Patient Outcomes
The patient will be free of urinary tract infection.

Nursing Interventions	Rationales
Monitor urinary output. Increase fluid intake unless contraindicated. Offer cranberry juice frequently. Measure intake and output.	Elderly people often voluntarily limit their fluid intake due to fear of incontinence. Additional fluids are necessary to dilute the urine. Cranberry juice acidifies the urine.
Offer nourishing foods of choice. Serve smaller, more frequent meals.	Adequate nutritional status is essential to recovery from infection. Appetite may improve if patient chooses foods and does not have to consume large amounts at one time.
Provide for frequent rest periods during the day.	Acute illness quickly devitalizes elderly persons.

▶ NURSING DIAGNOSIS: *Altered Thought Processes*

Related To delirium due to infectious process.

Defining Characteristics
- Disorientation
- Memory deficits

Patient Outcomes
The patient will
- remain oriented to time, place, and person.
- be protected from injury.

Nursing Interventions	Rationales
Monitor for signs of altered thought processes.	An acute infection can affect mental status in the elderly.
Implement reality orientation (RO) techniques.	Reality orientation techniques may be helpful in cases of temporary, reversible disorientation due to acute illness.
Implement fall prevention program.	Falls are a risk for the disoriented patient.
Assist to the bathroom q2h or as needed.	Falls frequently occur when a disoriented patient attempts to go to the bathroom.

▶ **NURSING DIAGNOSIS:** *High Risk for Infection (Septicemia)*

Risk Factors
- Urinary tract infection
- Suppressed inflammatory response
- Chronic disease

Patient Outcomes
The patient will be free of septicemia.

Nursing Interventions	Rationales
Monitor for signs of septicemia: 1. chills 2. fever 3. increased exhaustion Atypical signs in the elderly are blunted fever response, altered thought processes, and tachycardia and tachypnea.	Elderly persons with urinary tract infections (particularly those with enterococci) have high risk for septicemia. If atypical symptoms are absent, treatment is delayed. Morbidity and mortality from asepsis are more likely among the elderly population.
Monitor for signs of septic shock: 1. cool, pale extremities 2. elevated lactate 3. oliguria	Septicemia can quickly progress to sepsis syndrome and septic shock.

Nursing Interventions	Rationales
4. altered mental status 5. hypotension	
Prepare for management of sepsis: 1. blood cultures 2. volume replacement 3. antibiotic therapy 4. monitor vital signs 5. hourly urine output 6. serum electrolytes	Diligent treatment and monitoring reduce the incidence of mortality from sepsis syndrome and septic shock.

▶ **NURSING DIAGNOSIS:** *Health-seeking Behaviors (Prevention of Urinary Tract Infections)*

Related To desire to avoid urinary tract infections.

Defining Characteristics
• Expressed desire to prevent urinary tract infections.

Patient Outcomes
The patient will verbalize knowledge of preventive measures for urinary tract infections.

Nursing Interventions	Rationales
Provide information on preventive measures: 1. Drink 8–10 glasses of fluid per day unless contraindicated. Include cranberry juice in fluid choices. 2. Empty the bladder completely q3–4h. 3. Empty the bladder before and after sexual intercourse, washing genital area thoroughly.	Fluids dilute the urine, decreasing irritation and the risk of infection. Cranberry juice acidifies the urine. Emptying the bladder decreases the risk of urethral contamination.
Advise to report signs and symptoms of urinary tract infection promptly.	Early treatment may prevent complications.

Nursing Interventions	Rationales
Instruct patient to finish medications for urinary tract infections as prescribed.	Patients frequently discontinue medication when clinical signs dissipate even though bacteria are still present in urine.
NOTE: Additional instructions for women follow. Wipe from front to back after urinating. Cleanse thoroughly after bowel movement.	This avoids contamination of urethra with vaginal or rectal bacteria.
Avoid vaginal sprays, douches, bubble baths, and colored toilet paper.	These items can cause vaginal irritation, leaving it more susceptible to infection.
Wear underwear made of cotton rather than synthetic fabrics.	Cotton allows for better air circulation, avoiding bacterial growth.

DISCHARGE PLANNING/CONTINUITY OF CARE
- Review preventive measures with patient/family.
- Review signs of urinary tract infection and reinforce need to report to primary caregiver.

--- **Clinical Clip** ---

Diagnosis of urinary tract infection for patients in long-term care facilities should be based not solely on laboratory data but also on clinical manifestations. Antibiotic therapy should not be prescribed to patients with asymptomatic bacteremia.

BIBLIOGRAPHY

Bender, B. S. (1992). Diagnosis and management of sepsis. *Geriatric Focus on Infectious Diseases, 2*(3), 6–7, 10.

Crossley, K. B. (1992). Approach to the seriously ill, febrile nursing home patient with probable bacteremia or septicemia. In R. J. Duma (Ed.). *Recognition and management of nursing home infections*. Bethesda, MD: National Foundation for Infectious Diseases.

Fraser, D. (1993). Patient assessment: Infection in the elderly. *Journal of Gerontological Nursing, 19*(7), 5–11.

Garibaldi, R. A. (1992). Approach to the diagnosis and management of urinary tract infections in nursing home patients. In *Recognition and management of nursing home infections*. Bethesda, MD: National Foundation for Infectious Diseases.

Endocrine Conditions

$\mathcal{D}$IABETES MELLITUS

$\mathbf{D}$iabetes mellitus is a disease of varying severity with many serious complications if not managed properly. Type I, insulin-dependent diabetes mellitus (IDDM), occurs most often in thin people under 30 years of age. Type II, non-insulin-dependent diabetes mellitus (NIDDM), has an insidious onset and is more common in people over 40 years of age who rarely present classic symptoms.

ETIOLOGIES
- Type I: Little or no insulin is produced in the islets of Langerhans. Islets are smaller or fewer in number.
- Type II: Islets are present but either do not produce adequate amounts of insulin or secretion is delayed. There may be diminished insulin sensitivity in receptor cells or excess fat causing cells to become insulin resistant.

CLINICAL MANIFESTATIONS
Insulin-dependent diabetes mellitus
- Frequent urination (polyuria)
- Excessive thirst (polydipsia)
- Unusual hunger (polyphagia)
- Rapid loss of weight
- Irritability
- Weakness and fatigue
- Nausea and vomiting

Non-insulin-dependent diabetes mellitus
- Family history of diabetes
- Overweight
- Fatigue and drowsiness
- Skin infections, slow healing
- Pruritus
- Blurred vision
- Tingling, numbness, and burning sensations in feet

CLINICAL/DIAGNOSTIC FINDINGS

- Fasting blood sugar (FBS) ≥140 mg/dL obtained on two or more occasions if other causes are ruled out
- Glucose tolerance test (GTT) ≥200 mg/dL from a 2-h sample and at least one other sample
- Two-hour postprandial plasma glucose ≥200 mg/dL on adults over age 60
- Glycosated hemoglobin: test measures three minor hemoglobins—A_{1a}, A_{1b}, A_{1c}. If more than 8% of total hemoglobin within a RBC is A_{1c} the diabetes is not considered controlled.

▶ NURSING DIAGNOSIS: *Altered Nutrition—More Than Body Requirements*

Related To
- Decreased activity
- Lack of basic nutritional knowledge

Defining Characteristics
- Weight 20% over ideal for height and frame
- Triceps skin fold >15 mm in men, >25 mm in women
- Sedentary activity level

Patient Outcomes
The patient will
- maintain a steady weight loss of $\frac{1}{2}$ lb/week.
- strive to attain desirable body weight.
- reach and maintain satisfactory blood sugar levels.
- exercise daily and verbalize positive feelings about the effects of exercise.

Nursing Interventions

Assess patient's nutritional status:
1. Dietary intake
   - kinds and amounts of foods eaten each day
   - number of meals/snacks each day
   - time of day when meals/snacks are eaten
   - types of food that patient likes
2. Anthropometric measurements
   - height, weight
   - skinfold measurements
3. Biochemical measurements
   - serum albumin

Rationales

Lack of nutritional knowledge, poverty, isolation, decreased interest in eating, physical disability, and mental disorders are primary causes of malnutrition in the elderly. Drug-nutrient interactions are secondary causes. These causes result in a need for assistance with activities related to food consumption, such as shopping, meal preparation, and eating.

Nursing Interventions	Rationales

• transferrin
• hemoglobin
• hematocrit
4. Clinical evaluation
  • functional abilities/activities of daily living
  • mental status
5. Socioeconomic and environmental factors
  • financial resources
  • proximity to family/friends
  • alcohol or drug use	

Arrange for resources if necessary: 1. family/friends to shop and prepare meals 2. homemaker from a community agency to shop and prepare meals 3. delivery of meals-on-wheels 4. transportation to community senior center that serves meals at noon for elderly persons who enjoy socialization If financial resources are a problem, the charge for community services are based on income. Inquire into the Food Stamp Program funded by the federal government.	
Discuss the basics of healthy eating, pointing out the need to include items from each food group each day.	Elderly individuals are often not aware of their changing nutritional needs. Energy requirements decline from about 2,700 calories a day at age 30 to 2,100 calories a day by age 80. This is a result of a decline in basal energy metabolism and reduction in energy expenditures. Although caloric intake needs to be reduced, the nutritional value of food becomes more significant as eating habits affect the progress of many degenerative diseases associated with aging.

Nursing Interventions	Rationales
Explain the correlation between food intake and blood sugar levels.	Type II diabetes can frequently be controlled by dietary management. Insulin resistance decreases with weight loss and results in decreased hepatic glucose production and increased peripheral glucose uptake.
Discuss the principles of meal planning: 1. Maintain balanced nutrition and control portion sizes. 2. Eat at regular meal times. 3. Limit fat to ≤30% of total calories. 4. Plan for major portion of calories to be obtained from carbohydrates (55–60% of total calories), with emphasis on unrefined carbohydrates with fiber. 5. Maintain protein intake to 12–20% of total calories. 6. Restrict foods/beverages with concentrated sucrose. 7. Limit cholesterol intake to ≤300 mg/day. 8. Increase fiber intake. 9. Limit sodium intake to ≤3,000 mg/day. 10. Limit alcohol to ≤1–2 equivalents one to two times per week.	The goals of dietary management are to maintain adequate nutritional status, attain/maintain desirable body weight, and control blood glucose. NOTE: Whether restriction of dietary fat to ≤30% is desirable is controversial for Type II diabetes because of susceptibility to develop or worsen hypertriglyceridemia. This is not a problem if calories are also restricted. When diets are isocaloric, carbohydrates must also be increased.
Ask patient to keep a diary of daily food intake.	A food diary helps identify and prioritize problem areas that require alteration. It is best to suggest change gradually and to avoid change if preferences can be assimilated into the dietary management plan without risk of increasing blood glucose levels.
Assist patient to develop a personal exercise plan, taking into account physical condition, mental status, resources and interests. The patient	Regular exercise and endurance training lower triglycerides and blood glucose. After 5–10 min of exercise, glucose uptake from the

Nursing Interventions	Rationales
will need specific guidance and goals such as walking a certain distance each day. Consultation with the physician may be required.	blood is 7–20 times the resting rate, depending on how strenuous the exercise is. With regular exercise, weight loss will occur without severe caloric restrictions.
Monitor blood glucose levels at regular intervals at physician's office or laboratory: fasting blood or plasma glucose as recommended by physician and glycosylated hemoglobin assay (HbA_{1c}) 2/year recommended for stable type II diabetes.	Blood glucose levels done intermittently are useful in determining the need for dietary changes, oral hypoglycemic agents, or insulin. The HbA_{1c} is the single most accurate, objective assay for glycemic status. It measures average level of glucose over preceding 2–3 months. Self-monitoring of blood glucose (SMBG) has not been demonstrated to be useful or necessary in the management of diet-treated Type II diabetes. For Type II diabetic patients taking insulin or oral hypoglycemic agents, SMBG is recommended before breakfast or before dinner.
Tell patient to report to physician any signs of acute illness such as fever, nausea, vomiting, or signs of respiratory tract infections. Teach patient the cause, symptoms, and treatment of the diabetic emergencies, hypoglycemia and hyperglycemic hyperosmolar coma (HHC). (See Tables 20.1 and 20.2, pages 199–200.)	Anyone taking glucose-lowering agents, especially insulin or long-acting oral hypoglycemics, is at risk for hypoglycemia. Liver or renal impairment (common in elderly) increases the risk since insulin and oral hypoglycemic agents are metabolized in the liver and excreted by the kidneys. Alcohol, anabolic steroids, beta-adrenergic blockers, sulfonamides, and salicylates (>4 g/day) can decrease blood glucose levels or increase the effect of glucose-lowering agents. Hypoglycemia has a rapid onset and requires immediate treatment. Hyperglycemic hyperosmolar coma occurs predominantly in adults over 50 years and almost exclusively in patients with Type II

Nursing Interventions	Rationales
	diabetes. It develops most often in persons with undiagnosed diabetes, those with infections, and persons on diuretics. Onset may be insidious and prompt treatment is required.

▶ NURSING DIAGNOSIS: *High Risk for Impaired Skin Integrity*

Risk Factors
• Alterations in nutritional state
• Altered metabolic state
• Altered circulation

Patient Outcomes
The patient will
• be free of skin impairments.
• verbalize ability to care for skin and feet.
• identify reportable symptoms.

Nursing Interventions	Rationales
Advise patient to bathe or shower every other day using superfatted soap and moisturizer to keep the skin lubricated. Avoid using bubble bath, feminine hygiene sprays, or scented soaps. Tell patient to give special attention to skin folds and genital area to prevent fungal infections.	Changes in the skin associated with aging cause the skin to break down easily. This risk, in combination with diabetes, increases the risk for skin impairment resulting from infections and ulcerations. NOTE: Diabetic dermopathy is common in older diabetics and is caused by diabetic changes in the small blood vessels. These light brown, scaly patches may be mistaken for "age spots." They are usually noted on the lower legs but are not symmetrical. The patches do not hurt, itch, or ulcerate and require no treatment.

Nursing Interventions	Rationales
Teach the need for regular foot care. Instruct patient to wash feet daily in lukewarm water and mild soap and to rinse thoroughly and pat dry. Give special attention to the areas between the toes. Inspect both feet, using a mirror and light for the soles if necessary. Look for signs of injury or infection: blisters, ulcers, fissures, or reddened areas; red or purple discolorations on the lower legs; temperature changes; absence of hair growth; or thick, deformed toenails. Advise patient to notify physician if these signs appear. Apply moisturizer sparingly. Instruct patient to never cut or pick at corns, calluses, splinters, blisters, or abscesses. Chemicals and medications should not be used on the feet without a physician's order. Wear well-fitting shoes and avoid going barefoot.	Foot care is important for elderly diabetics because peripheral circulation is generally impaired. Any injury of the lower extremities will therefore be slow to heal and presents a risk of infection that can lead to ulcers and eventually gangrene.
Teach patient to trim and file toenails after soaking in warm water for 15–20 min or after a bath or shower. Use a toenail clipper to cut them a little at a time instead of cutting the entire nail with one clip. Follow the curve of the toe. The nail length should be even with the ends of the toes. Refer to podiatrist if necessary.	Proper nail care is necessary to avoid accidental injury to the feet, causing infection and eventually gangrene. Nails become thicker and more brittle with aging, making nail care more difficult. If the patient also has mobility problems, it may be preferable to obtain the services of the podiatrist.
Instruct patient to avoid the use of heating pads or hot water bottles.	There may be reduced sensation in the lower extremities and thermal injuries may not be noted by the patient.
Advise patient that a pillow placed at the end of the bed will keep the covers off the feet. Avoid wearing round garters or tying knots to keep stockings up. Instruct patient to	Avoid situations that further compromise circulation.

Nursing Interventions	Rationales
avoid sitting with legs crossed or standing in one position for a long time. If patient uses tobacco, refer to a smoking cessation program.	
Advise wearing seamless cotton or wool socks, changing daily. Well-fitting panty hose can be worn for short periods of time. Shoes should be $\frac{1}{2}$ in. longer than the longest toe and wide enough to avoid squeezing the toes. Leather or canvas shoes with firm soles and soft uppers are the best choice. Avoid sandals or open-toed shoes. Break new shoes in by wearing them for no more than 2 h the first few times. Allow shoes to "rest" 12–24 h between wearing.	Cotton and wool absorb moisture better than synthetic fabrics. Improperly fitting footwear can cause pressure, resulting in impaired skin integrity.

▶ NURSING DIAGNOSIS: *High Risk for Visual Alterations*

Risk Factors
- Hyperglycemia and consequent damage to retinal blood vessels

Patient Outcomes
The patient will
- strive to maintain blood glucose control.
- arrange for regular ophthalmological eye examinations.
- recognize and report signs/symptoms of impaired vision.

Nursing Interventions	Rationales
Advise patient to have an eye examination once a year with a funduscope, which requires that pupils be dilated.	The examiner must be able to observe the blood vessels on the retina to fully assess the condition of the eyes.
Advise to report at once symptoms of blurred vision, "cobwebs,"	These symptoms could indicate blood vessel abnormalities on the

Nursing Interventions	Rationales
"floaters," or sudden loss of vision (see Sensory Impairments, Vision, page 283).	retina, leading to diabetic retinopathy.
Request kidney function tests if there is evidence of retinopathy.	Diabetic nephropathy does not occur in the absence of retinopathy.

▶ **NURSING DIAGNOSIS:** *High Risk for Altered Tissue Perfusion (Cardiovascular)*

Risk Factors
- Coronary atherosclerosis
- Age >40 years
- Concurrent hypertension
- Smoking
- Obesity
- Hyperlipidemia
- Dislipidemia

Patient Outcomes
The patient will
- strive to maintain blood glucose control.
- make necessary life-style changes to reduce the risk of cardiovascular disease.
- arrange for regular blood pressure monitoring and laboratory tests.

Nursing Interventions	Rationales
Provide instruction to assist patient to reduce risk factors: 1. smoking cessation classes 2. dietary reduction of fat, cholesterol, and calories if necessary 3. exercise plan 4. explain need for compliance with medication regime	Reducing risk factors may prevent cardiovascular disease.
Discuss with patient the warning signs of heart attack, stroke, and hypertension. Check available community resources to see if free blood pressure monitoring is available to the elderly on a regular basis.	Recognition of signs and symptoms and early treatment may be life-saving actions.

▶ NURSING DIAGNOSIS: *High Risk for Altered Tissue Perfusion (Kidney)*

Risk Factors
- Poor blood glucose control
- Genetic predisposition to diabetic nephropathy
- Systemic hypertension

Patient Outcomes
The patient will
- strive to maintain blood glucose control.
- arrange for regular monitoring of blood pressure.
- identify measures to prevent urinary tract infections.
- recognize signs/symptoms of urinary tract problems.
- arrange for regular monitoring of kidney function tests.

Nursing Interventions	Rationales
Teach patient the function of the kidneys and preventive measures for urinary tract infections (see Urinary Tract Infections, page 182).	Infections of the urinary tract increase the risk of kidney disease. Persons who become diabetics before age 40 and who are insulin dependent are at special risk for developing kidney problems associated with diabetes. Type II patients have a much lower risk but should be aware of the possible risk and need for prompt treatment for urinary tract disorders.
Teach the patient the signs/symptoms of urinary tract infections.	Early treatment may prevent further disease of the urinary tract.
Check blood urea nitrogen (BUN) and serum creatinine regularly.	These tests evaluate renal function. The serum creatinine is a more specific test. An elevated BUN, especially in the elderly, does not necessarily indicate kidney disease. Serum creatinine is more reliable because kidney impairment is virtually the only cause of elevated levels.
Suggest that a routine urinalysis be completed when patient has blood glucose drawn.	If routine urinalysis indicates presence of white blood cells and/or bacteria, request a culture and

Nursing Interventions	Rationales
	sensitivity for treatment of bladder infection. Proteinuria is an indication of diabetic nephropathy but may also be a sign of other diseases.
Monitor drugs excreted through kidneys.	Initially, drug-induced renal dysfunction may occur before it is noted in the BUN and serum creatinine.

▶ NURSING DIAGNOSIS: *High Risk for Peripheral Neurovascular Dysfunction*

Risk Factors
- Height
- Male sex
- Age
- Hypertension
- Duration of diabetes
- Glucose control
- Cholesterol level
- Smoking

Patient Outcomes
The patient will
- maintain blood glucose control.
- avoid alcohol and other chemical toxins.
- implement measures to prevent foot injuries.

Nursing Interventions	Rationales
Discuss need for preventive measures: 1. Maintain blood glucose control (see page 191). 2. Avoid alcohol and other chemical toxins. 3. Prevent foot injuries (see page 193).	Ignoring these measures may trigger the onset of neuropathy or hasten its progression.
Tell patient to report abnormal sensations in lower extremities: dull, aching, burning, lancinating, or	These symptoms suggest diabetic neuropathy but may also be indicative of other diseases which

Nursing Interventions	Rationales
crushing pain and paresthesia (tingling, burning, coldness, and numbness).	need to be excluded before a diagnosis is made.
Evaluate yearly for peripheral neuropathy including these exams: 1. pinprick 2. proprioception 3. reflexes, deep tendon 4. two-point discrimination 5. light touch	Peripheral neuropathies are not always initially painful so the patient may not recognize and report clinical manifestations.
Suggest consultation with health care professional familiar with diabetic painful neuropathy if symptoms are present.	Treatment is required and should be directed toward the specific type of peripheral nerve pain: 1. hyperesthesia: pain caused by contact with objects that normally do not cause pain (clothing, bedding) 2. paresthesia: sensations of constant tingling 3. dysethesia: sensations of pins and needles, painful numbness, intense burning 3. muscle pain: dull, achy night cramps, shooting pains
Assess ambulation skill.	Decreased proprioception frequently occurs with diabetic neuropathy, resulting in ataxic gait and unsteadiness.
If there is evidence of decreased proprioception, teach patient to 1. adopt a wider gait. 2. use a handrail when climbing stairs. 3. use vision to compensate for proprioception loss. 4. keep a night light on at home, always have a flashlight available, and avoid the need to walk in dark areas.	These safety measures may prevent injury resulting from falling.

DISCHARGE PLANNING/CONTINUITY OF CARE

- Evaluate effectiveness of patient teaching. Reinforce instruction if necessary.
- Make referrals if necessary for community services:
  - home health nurse
  - homemaker
  - home-delivered meals
- Provide information for the following:
  - community classes on diabetes
  - consultation with dietician if necessary
  - obtaining services of podiatrist
  - obtaining services of ophthalmologist
- Provide information for the following:
  - follow-up laboratory tests
  - blood pressure monitoring if home health nurse will not be monitoring patient's status

---

Clinical Clip

Results of the Diabetes Control and Complications Trial (DCCT) indicate that tight blood glucose control can be obtained with intensive insulin therapy if the patient is highly motivated and can implement appropriate life-style management.

Table 20.1 • Hypoglycemia

Causes

Overdose of antidiabetic agents
Reduced food intake and usual dosage of antidiabetic agent

Signs and Symptoms

Sweating, clamminess	Hunger, anxiety, headache
Tremors	Unusual behavior
Rapid pulse and respirations	Poor coordination
Unconsciousness	

Treatment: Any of These

4 oz orange juice or apple juice	1 tbsp jelly
3 oz nondiet cola	2 packets sugar
7–9 hard candies	4 sugar cubes
OR	

Commercial glucose products or glycogen

Table 20.1 • *continued*

This treatment brings only temporary improvement. Follow with longer acting carbohydrates such as crackers, milk, or high-fiber fruit to avoid recurrence.

NOTE: Some medications may mask tachycardia and sweating such as beta blockers, clonidine, quanethidine, and reserpine. Monitor blood glucose levels closely if patient begins or stops taking these medications.

Table 20.2 • Hyperglycemic Hyperosmolar Coma

Causes

Untreated or poorly controlled diabetes mellitus
Can be triggered by infection, extreme emotional stress, blood-sugar-raising drugs, surgery, myocardial infarction

Signs and Symptoms

Extreme dehydration with serum osmolarity elevated >350 mOsm/L
Blood glucose >600 mg/dL
Lethargy, confusion, depressed sensorium, unconsciousness, rapid pulse, respirations, warm, flushed, dry, loose skin, soft eyeballs

Treatment

Fluid and electrolyte replacement
Insulin
Advise patient to purchase Medic-Alert® device

BIBLIOGRAPHY

Ahmed, F. E. (1992). Effect of nutrition on the health of the elderly. *Journal of the American Dietetic Association, 92*(9), 1102–1108.

Diabetes update. (1993). *Nursing 93, 23*(8), 59–61.

Lebovitz, H. E. (Ed.). (1991). *Therapy for diabetes mellitus and related disorders.* Alexandria, VA: American Diabetes Association.

Murray, R. (1993). Home before dark. *American Journal of Nursing, 93*(11), 36–42.

Needham, J. F. (1993). *Gerontological nursing, a restorative approach.* Albany, NY: Delmar.

Thom, S. L. (1992). Nutritional management of the elderly client with diabetes. *The Dialogue, 1*(3), 1–3, 7.

Neurological Conditions

ᴀʟZHEIMER'S DISEASE AND RELATED DEMENTIAS

Alzheimer's disease (AD) is an organic mental disorder classified as one of several forms of dementia. Dementia is a clinical syndrome characterized by the loss of intellectual functioning (Table 21.1, page 217). Sixty percent of all dementias are due to AD. The onset usually occurs after age 65 and affects more women than men. The disease is progressive and irreversible, with insidious onset and no regard for race, color, sex, socioeconomic status, intellectual level, or occupation. Nerve filaments accumulate within the nerve cell, forming neurofibrillary tangles. Plaques consisting of neuronal breakdown products are deposited outside the cell. These plaques contain a protein fragment, amyloid beta-protein. Persons with AD also have decreased levels of acetylcholine, a neurotransmitter. The areas of the brain producing this chemical are thought to be the source of the problem.

ETIOLOGIES
The cause of AD remains unknown. Current theories include research in
- the role of amyloid proteins in the brain.
- the possibility of a slow-acting virus that triggers a reaction causing AD.
- a genetic link.
- an autoimmune reaction associated with antibodies found in the plaques.
- toxins due to the presence of excess accumulation of aluminum in the plaques.

CLINICAL MANIFESTATIONS
The individual with AD progresses through several stages of mental and physical deterioration which may occur rapidly or may proceed slowly over a number of years:
- loss of short-term memory and eventually of long-term memory
- decreasing attention span and increasing distractibility

- impaired judgment
- loss of impulse control
- changes in affect
- confabulation
- difficulty in making decisions, plans
- loss of abilities in reading, writing, arithmetic
- disorientation to time, place, and eventually person
- wandering and pacing
- aphasia
- perceptual deficits including agnosia, apraxia, perseveration
- rummaging and hoarding
- agitation, anxiety, and catastrophic reactions
- delusions and hallucinations
- sundowning
- hyerorality
- eventually total dependence and incontinence

CLINICAL/DIAGNOSTIC FINDINGS

There are no specific diagnostic tests for AD. Diagnostic procedures are used to rule out the following:
- delirium (acute confusion) associated with metabolic disturbances, cardiovascular and cerebral vascular disorders, trauma, infections, alcohol intoxication, or withdrawal
- depression (pseudodementia)
- other dementias

These diagnostic measures are completed to rule out other diseases which may have similar symptoms. These test results are nonspecific for Alzheimer's and most other dementias but will detect other diseases that have similar symptoms but which may be reversible:
- blood studies: electrolyte and metabolic panel, thyroid function tests, complete blood count, vitamin B_{12} and folate levels, tests for syphilis and human immunodeficiency virus (HIV)
- electrocardiogram (EKG) and electroencephalogram (EEG)
- magnetic resonance imaging (MRI) and positive emission tomography (PET)

These examinations may identify the clinical manifestations listed above:
- history and physical examination
- psychiatric and neuropsychological examinations
- mental status examination (*See* Appendix D, page 349.)

▶ NURSING DIAGNOSIS: *Altered Thought Processes*

Related To progressive neuronal degeneration, resulting in disruption of the thought processes that link feelings to actions.

Defining Characteristics

- Memory deficits
- Impaired judgment
- Impulsivity
- Misinterpretation of the environment
- Distractibility
- Delusions and hallucinations

Patient Outcomes

The patient will remain calm and avoid experiencing agitation and anxiety that result from the altered thought processes.

Nursing Interventions	Rationales
Assess orientation by asking, "What are your plans today?"	Asking questions the patient cannot answer such as "Do you know what day it is today?" causes frustration leading to agitation and increases feelings of worthlessness. Asking the open-ended question does not require a specific answer from the patient. The answer is an indication of the patient's orientation. For some patients, answering an open-ended question may be stressful. Utilize such questions only when it is necessary to assess orientation.
Facilitate orientation in early stages: 1. Provide large clocks and calendars with easy-to-read numbers. 2. Open the window blinds or drapes during the day. 3. Provide environmental clues such as seasonal decorations. 4. Place signs in appropriate places such as the picture of a toilet on the bathroom door.	These are helpful reminders in the early stage of the disease. The cues assist in orientation to time and place and prolong physical independence. NOTE: Reality orientation is inappropriate during the middle and later stages of the disease. It is pointless and frustrating to the patient and caregivers to expect the patient to remain oriented.
Arrange a therapeutic environment: 1. Provide adequate nonglare lighting. 2. Hang only artwork that is familiar, such as landscapes and seascapes.	Environmental misperceptions may result from shadows, poor lighting, abstract artwork, or stressful television programs. Seeing one's image in a mirror may be frightening when the

Nursing Interventions	**Rationales**
3. Use nonglare glass on pictures. 4. Pull blinds or draw draperies after dark. 5. Monitor television viewing. 6. Remove mirrors from the area. 7. Maintain a quiet, stable environment.	patient thinks it is another person advancing. Noise can be over-stimulating, causing anxiety and agitation. To the person with a dementia, change is intolerable.
Attend to feelings rather than the behavior: "I know it bothers you," when patient has delusions. Avoid reasoning or using logic to explain the false idea. Overlook the delusion without reinforcing it if the patient is content. If the delusion causes anxiety, reassure and stay with the patient. Moving the patient to a quieter environment may be helpful.	A delusion is very real to the patient and may be based on experiences from the past. In later stages of the disease, the patient may be happier rocking her "babies" than she is in present-day reality. Accept the patient where he or she is at the moment to increase feelings of self-worth. An attempt to change the patient's thoughts can result in a catastrophic reaction.
Monitor behavior if hallucinations are present. Use reassurance. Psychotropic medication is warranted for the prevention of hallucinations or delusions that are disturbing the patient.	Hallucinations (and delusions) can result in disruptive behavior that may be dangerous to the patient, other patients, or staff.

▶ NURSING DIAGNOSIS: *High Risk for Trauma*

Risk Factors
- Wandering behavior
- Inability to recognize sensory cues for danger
- Impaired judgment
- Impulsivity
- Memory deficits

Patient Outcomes
The patient will remain free of serious injury while retaining as much independence and freedom of movement as possible.

Nursing Interventions	Rationales
Avoid the use of chemical or physical restraints to prevent wandering. Allow wandering by maintaining safe environment (see below). Obtain a Medic-Alert® bracelet. Keep an up-to-date snapshot available and monitor patient's clothing. For institutional setting install an alarm system that is triggered when patient exits building.	The use of restraints hastens mental and physical deterioration and increases feelings of frustration, hostility, and distrust. Identification is necessary in case the patient gets lost.
Maintain a safe environment: 1. Place bed in low position, removing wheels if necessary, and set the brakes. 2. Evaluate the need for siderails. The risk of injury is often greater with siderails. 3. Arrange furniture to allow for unobstructed walking and remove clutter. 4. Anchor rugs and electrical wires. 5. Place nonslip mat in tub and install handgrip. 6. Lock up smoking materials, sharp objects, power tools, chemicals, and guns. 7. Place a cover over the thermostat. 8. Lower the temperature of the water heater. 9. Lock the controls of the stove. 10. Remove poisonous plants, chemicals, and cleaning supplies from the environment.	Adapt the environment to the needs and current behaviors of the patient. The patient can move about the room(s) freely, avoiding frustration.
Monitor for signs of fatigue. If present, walk with the patient toward a chair or bed and show the patient how to sit or lie down.	It is unknown why persons with AD wander. It may be because they forget how to find a chair or how to sit down. They may not experience the feelings normally associated with fatigue.

▶ NURSING DIAGNOSIS: *Sleep Pattern Disturbance*

Related To sundowning.

Defining Characteristics
- Awake at times when sleep would normally occur
- Restlessness
- Increased disorientation
- Agitation

Patient Outcomes
The patient will
- sleep for longer periods of time.
- experience less agitation if awake at inappropriate times.

Nursing Interventions	Rationales
Assess patient's sleep-wake pattern.	Assessing the pattern may indicate that the patient needs to be kept awake during the day with more activities or the patient may not be napping during the day and thus becomes overfatigued and unable to sleep at night. In this case, a short nap early in the afternoon may be beneficial.
Ask family about patient's previous sleep habits and bedtime routine.	Following the patient's usual routine may facilitate sleep. Examples: wearing socks to bed, wearing pajamas instead of a nightgown or vice versa, using two pillows, sleeping with the window open, going to sleep with the radio/TV on, drinking warm milk or a glass of wine at bedtime, or having a nightlight.
Implement a consistent bedtime routine: 1. Allow patient ample time for toileting. 2. Avoid television viewing or stimulating activities prior to bedtime. 3. Assist the patient in simple exercises (active range of motion) 1 h before bedtime.	Consistency in caregivers, routine, and environment is the key to successful care of patients with AD. It promotes feelings of trust and relieves anxiety associated with unpredictability. Attention to physical needs enhances comfort and promotes relaxation.

Nursing Interventions

4. Provide an easy-to-chew, easy-to-digest, noncaffeinated snack.
5. Assist the patient to take a warm bath and to do oral care.
6. Give a slow backrub.
7. Implement strategies recommended by the family.

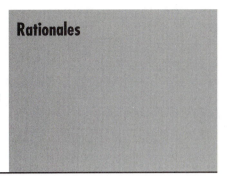

▶ **NURSING DIAGNOSIS:** *Functional Incontinence*

Related To lack of awareness of need to void and inability to find the bathroom.

Defining Characteristics
• Loss of urine before reaching the bathroom

Patient Outcomes
The patient will
• remain dry in between toileting.
• urinate in the toilet.

Nursing Interventions	Rationales
In early stages of disease: 1. Place a picture of a toilet on the bathroom door. 2. Remind/take to the bathroom q2h on a consistent schedule. Provide comfort and privacy. Praise the patient if he or she is dry at toileting time. Praise if patient urinates in toilet.	Retraining is not an appropriate intervention for persons with dementia. The goal is to keep the patient dry by toileting at regular times throughout the day. In the later stages, incontinent pads will be needed as bladder control becomes less stable.

▶ **NURSING DIAGNOSIS:** *Anxiety*

Related To
• Delusions
• Hallucinations
• Perceptual deficits
• Overstimulating environment

Defining Characteristics
- Increased motor activity: pacing, agitation, irritability
- Verbalizations become louder and more frequent
- Striking out at others
- Refusal to participate in activities of daily living

Patient Outcomes
The patient will
- be relieved of anxiety, as evidenced by decreased motor activity and verbalizations.
- be free from catastrophic reactions.

Nursing Interventions	Rationales
Assess the situation when signs of anxiety are evident: 1. environment: noise, lighting, numbers of people in area, amount of activity, changes in routine 2. caregivers: unsure of their abilities, inadequate numbers, low tolerance levels for behaviors	Environmental conditions can create anxiety due to noise, activity, and frequent changes in lighting. Patients with AD can "read" the people around them. They may read the anxiety, tension, or dislike in a caregiver's body language and respond accordingly.
Maintain a calm environment: 1. Reduce the noise level by controlling the use of radios and televisions. 2. Avoid the use of intercoms and install telephones that light instead of ring for incoming calls. 3. Avoid abrupt intrusions into the patient's personal space. 4. Touch the patient only after he or she is aware of your presence.	Patients with AD are unable to tolerate constant noise and confusion in the environment. They respond by becoming increasingly anxious. Clusters of people may cause the patient to become suspicious, thinking he or she will be attacked. Although many patients with AD tend to "cling," they generally do not respond well to the sudden and unpredictable closeness of another person.
Evaluate these factors if patient experiences catastrophic reaction: 1. When did incident happen? For example, during meal time or bath time? 2. What behavior was observed? Description needs to be objective and explicit, i.e., "struck NA's	Careful evaluation may reveal a trigger for the incident. Avoiding its reoccurrence will prevent future catastrophic reactions. Documenting only the patient's behavior does not provide sufficient data to identify the cause of the problem. All behavior has a reason, and for

Nursing Interventions

hand when she attempted to feed patient."
3. Where did behavior occur?
4. Who else was present and what were they doing?
5. What else was happening at the time?
6. Who were the caregivers and how did caregivers respond to the behavior?
7. How did patient react?

Rationales

persons with AD, catastrophic reactions may result from an over-stimulating environment, from inappropriate staff actions, from anxiety related to care, or from internal stress related to infections or other physical illness.

▶ NURSING DIAGNOSIS: *Impaired Verbal Communication*

Related To destruction of brain cells.

Defining Characteristics
- Difficulty expressing thoughts verbally
- Difficulty in comprehending others

Patient Outcomes
The patient will
- be understood by caregivers.
- display fewer episodes of frustration related to impaired communication.

Nursing Interventions

Facilitate communication by
1. engaging in conversation in a place free of noise and distractions.
2. speaking at eye level and main-taining eye contact.
3. using gentle touch but avoiding getting too close.
4. speaking slowly, softly, using short, simple sentences, and giving time to comprehend and respond.
5. using patient's word substitutions if they are consistent.

Rationales

Persons with AD will not regain the use of language once it is lost. Caregivers need to be aware of the patient's abilities and adapt their communication techniques accordingly.

Nursing Interventions

6. utilizing humor and laughter as a means of communication.
7. showing respect for feelings.
8. relying on use of facial expressions and gestures as comprehension skills diminish.
9. considering negative behaviors a method of communication when verbal skills are lost.

Rationales

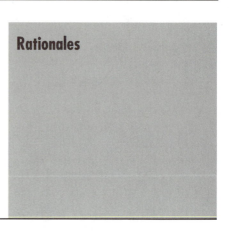

▶ **NURSING DIAGNOSIS:** *High Risk for Altered Nutrition—Less Than Body Requirements*

Risk Factors

- Shortened attention span
- Apraxia
- Agnosia
- Energy expenditures used for wandering

Patient Outcomes
The patient will maintain usual body weight.

Nursing Interventions	Rationales
Toilet before each meal. Position patient close to table with feet flat on the floor.	Provide for physical comfort.
Prepare food before placing it in front of patient: cutting meat, pouring beverages, seasoning the food, etc. Place Dycem or wet washcloth under plate to avoid slipping. Attach a guard to the plate; fill cups and glasses only partially.	Make eating as simple as possible to avoid frustration.
Use plain dishes without a pattern. Place only one course at a time in front of the patient. Remove all condiments from the table. Eliminate	Avoid sources of confusion that will distract the patient from eating.

Nursing Interventions	Rationales
environmental distractions. Turn off the radio or television. Move to a quieter area if other persons in dining area are noisy.	
Check food temperatures, especially if food was warmed in a microwave.	Avoid burns from hot food.
Maintain a position of slight head flexion for eating. Use a commercial thickener for fluids if necessary.	Avoid aspiration while eating.
Assist the patient by placing a glass or utensil in hand and give brief, simple instructions, using hand-over-hand techniques. Moisten lips and give small amount of fluid to swallow. If perseveration is noted, gently touch the cheek or lips with a finger and instruct the patient to swallow.	Eliminate the problems associated with perceptual deficits such as agnosia, apraxia, latency, and perseveration.

▶ **NURSING DIAGNOSIS:** *Self-Care Deficits (Grooming and Hygiene)*

Related To
- Memory loss
- Shortened attention span
- Apraxia
- Agnosia

Defining Characteristics
- Inability to recognize items required for grooming and hygiene
- Inability to use items required for grooming and hygiene
- Inability to remember instructions
- Inability to attend to task long enough to complete it

Patient Outcomes
The patient will complete activities of daily living (grooming and hygiene) with minimal assistance. (As the disease progresses, the amount of assistance needed will increase until total care is required.)

Nursing Interventions	Rationales
Provide a set-up: Place items needed for a task in front of patient. Use verbal cues, hand-over-hand techniques, and demonstration to utilize patient's abilities. Example: Prepare the toothbrush, hand it to patient, and say "please brush your teeth." Go through the motions if necessary or place it in patient's hand and assist guiding toothbrush to mouth. Instruct caregivers to avoid doing what the patient can do for self.	Once a skill is lost, it cannot be regained. However, independence may be prolonged if appropriate assistive techniques are utilized.
Observe for perseveration, for example, washing face over and over during bath. Gently take hand, praise patient's efforts, and direct hand to another part of the body.	Redirection is needed to complete the task.
Consider tub baths rather than showers. Check water and room temperature. Provide privacy but do not leave alone in bathtub.	Baths are frequently less threatening than showers and can be more relaxing.
Ask the family to provide clothing that is easy to manipulate, such as jogging suits, clothes with velcro closures, and front-opening dresses.	Maintain dressing skills as long as possible.
Arrange for regular appointments with barber or hair dresser. Help patient maintain attractive, well-groomed appearance.	Even though the patient is disoriented, self-esteem is still important.
Monitor oral care and examine mouth regularly if patient is taking phenytoin.	Phenytoin may be prescribed for seizures, which are often manifested in persons with AD. Phenytoin can cause swelling and overgrowth of gum tissue if meticulous oral care is not maintained.

▶ NURSING DIAGNOSIS: *Altered Family Processes*

Related To disruption in family relationships.

Defining Characteristics

Family members may be

- fatigued due to 24-h/day responsibilities.
- suffering feelings of guilt related to periodic frustration, resentment, and anger.
- worried about need for nursing home placement and financial needs.

Family Outcomes

The family will

- ventilate their feelings to an appropriate staff member.
- express a feeling of comfort with the decision to place their loved one in the facility.

Nursing Interventions	Rationales
Build a trusting relationship with the family and let them know there is a staff person(s) available to listen to their concerns.	The family needs to know that their feelings are acceptable and not unusual.
Invite and encourage the family's participation in the planning of care.	Family members have often cared for the patient for several years. They can share their ideas and provide valuable information. They will begin to know the staff and feel more comfortable and at ease.
Allow family members to participate in the care to the extent they wish to be involved. Assess the family's feelings and proceed accordingly.	Some families enjoy opportunities to continue to "do" for the patient without the ongoing responsibility they carried when the patient was at home. Others choose to relinquish the caregiving role.
Assess family's ideas regarding physical expressions of affection. If this is important to family, let them know that these actions are beneficial and appropriate. Provide privacy for visits (especially spousal visits).	Hugging and touching are positive methods of communication and can ease anxiety in both the patient and family members.
Assure the family that staff is not judging the patient by the behavior that is exhibited. Tell them that this is expected behavior in persons with AD.	Families are often embarrassed by the behavior and may try to deny the patient's problems.

Nursing Interventions	Rationales
Avoid being judgmental if family visits decrease. Assure them that appropriate care will be given in their absence and that they will be notified of any staff concerns. Encourage them to take respite to avoid emotional and physical exhaustion.	Some families find it difficult to cope when a loved one is steadily deteriorating. Each person must develop his or her own coping mechanisms without criticism from others. It is important to take time out for physical and emotional renewal.
Provide information for AD community support groups.	The family may find comfort in associating with others who are experiencing similar situations.

DISCHARGE PLANNING/CONTINUITY OF CARE

If the patient is in a long-term care facility, placement is probably considered permanent:

- Encourage family participation in care planning and care giving if appropriate.
- Monitor patient for signs of physical illness.
- Discuss advance directives with family.
- Provide information on local Alzheimer's support groups.

If the patient is at home:

- Provide family with information on community adult day care and/or respite care.
- Arrange for homemaker services to allow the primary caregiver brief periods of relief from responsibilities.
- Provide information on local Alzheimer's support groups.

Clinical Clip

Tacrine is a new medication approved for people diagnosed with AD who have mild to moderate cognitive impairment. Subtle changes in memory and attention span and increased motivation have been noted in studies. It has not been demonstrated to improve mood and behavior or to decrease agitation and sleep disturbances.

Table 21.1 • Overview of Major Forms of Dementia

Disease	Features	Major Clinical Manifestations	Course
Alzheimer's	Involvement of higher brain structures, neurofibrillary tangles, neuritic plaque	Memory deficits, disorientation, cognitive impairment, wandering, aphasia	Onset: 60–80, slowly progressive
Multi-infarct dementia	Multiple cerebral infarctions	Emotional lability, dysarthria, dysphasia, seizures, cognitive impairment	Onset: 55–70, outcome depends on rate of new lesions occurring
Huntington's	Autosomal dominant disorder	Choreiform movements, dysarthria, dysphagia	Onset: 25–45, average duration 15 years
Parkinson's	Deficiency of dopamine	Movement disorders, dysarthria, dysphagia, psychotic symptoms	Onset: 55–60, several years duration
Creutzfeldt-Jakob	Noninflammatory virus, spongiform changes in brain	Cognitive impairment, myoclonus, extrapyramidal movements	Onset: 50–60, rapidly progressive
Pick's	Shrinkage of localized areas	Cognitive impairment, depression, apathy, wandering, disorientation	Onset >70, average of 4 years duration
Syphilis	Spirochete	Cognitive impairment, tremors, ataxia, dysarthria	Paresis 15–20 years > primary infection
Gerstmann-Strausler-Scheinker	Noninflammatory virus, spongiform changes	Cerebellar ataxia, cognitive impairment	Slowly progressive
Kuru	Spongiform changes	Cerebellar ataxia, cognitive impairment, clonus, malaise	Death within 12 months
Acquired immunodeficiency syndrome dementia	HIV-1 infection	Ataxia, tremors, hypertonia, paraparesis, myoclonus, apathy	Symptoms sometimes precede diagnosis of systemic AIDS

Table 21.2 • Diagnostic Criteria for Dementia*

A. Impairment in short- and long-term memory

B. At least one of the following:
1. Impairment in abstract thinking
2. Impaired judgment
3. Other disturbances of higher cortical function such as aphasia, apraxia, agnosia, and constructional difficulty
4. Personality change, i.e., alteration or accentuation of premorbid traits

C. The disturbance in A and B significantly interferes with work or usual social activities or relationships with others

D. Not occurring exclusively during the course of delirium

E. Either 1 or 2:
1. There is evidence from the history, physical examination, or laboratory tests of a specific organic factor(s) judged to be etiologically related to the disturbance
2. In the absence of such evidence, an etiologic organic factor can be presumed if the disturbance cannot be accounted for by any nonorganic mental disorder, e.g., major depression accounting for cognitive impairment

See Appendix D, Mini Mental Status Examination, page 349.
From Diagnostic and Statistical Manual of Mental Disorder, *3rd ed., rev. (1987). Washington, DC: American Psychiatric Association.*

BIBLIOGRAPHY

Algase, D. L. (1992). A century of progress: Today's strategies for responding to wandering behavior. *Journal of Gerontological Nursing, 18*(11), 28–34.

American Psychiatric Association. (1987). *Diagnostic and Statistical Manual of Mental Disorders,* 3rd ed., rev. Washington, DC: American Psychiatric Association.

Foreman, M. D., & Grabowski, R. (1992). Diagnostic dilemma: Cognitive impairment of the elderly. *Journal of Gerontological Nursing, 18*(9), 5–12.

Mace, N., & Rabins, P. (1991). *The 36-hour day,* 2nd ed. Baltimore, MD: Johns Hopkins Press.

Namazi, K. H., & Johnson, B. D. (1992). Pertinent autonomy for residents with dementias: Modification of the physical environment to enhance independence. *American Journal of Alzheimer's Disease and Related Disorders & Research, Jan./Feb.,* vol. 7, 16–21.

Needham, J. F. (1993). *Gerontological nursing, a restorative approach.* Albany, NY: Delmar.

Ryden, M. B., & Feldt, K. S. (1992). Goal-directed care: Caring for aggressive nursing home residents with dementia. *Journal of Gerontological Nursing, 18*(11), 35–41.

CEREBROVASCULAR ACCIDENT (STROKE)

A stroke (CVA) usually results from progressive disease developed over a long period of time but rarely detected in routine physical examinations. The underlying disease process may be hypertension, blood vessel disease, impaired cardiac function, autoimmune disease, or a disturbance in the blood-clotting mechanism. Transient ischemic attack (TIA) may provide warning signs that stroke is imminent (see Transient Ischemic Attack, page 107). The consequences of stroke are devastating, with symptoms dependent on the location and extent of brain damage.

ETIOLOGIES
- Thrombus
- Embolus
- Hemorrhage

CLINICAL MANIFESTATIONS
Vary depending on the extent and location of ischemia and the degree of spontaneous recovery that has occurred:
- motor impairments
- communication disorders
- sensory/perceptual/spatial alterations
- cognitive impairments
- emotional effects

CLINICAL/DIAGNOSTIC FINDINGS
- Computerized tomography (CT) scan: cerebral infarct
- Hemorrhage, arteriovenous malformation
- Lumbar puncture: increased pressure, bloody cerebrospinal fluid
- Cerebral angiography: occlusion or narrowing of large vessels

▶ NURSING DIAGNOSIS: *Impaired Physical Mobility*

Related To
- Hemiplegia
- Spasticity
- Diminished endurance

Defining Characteristics
- Inability to move extremities on affected side
- Decreased strength and endurance

Patient Outcomes
The patient will
- maintain current levels of range of motion (ROM) in all joints.
- remain free of contractures.
- transfer independently.
- ambulate with a quad cane.

NOTE: The last two outcomes may not be realistic for all patients. Some may permanently require assistance with transfer whereas others may need to be transferred with a mechanical lifter. Some may never ambulate, but be able to propel their own wheelchairs.

Nursing Interventions	Rationales
Establish schedule for repositioning at least q2h. 1. Assess for presence of synergy patterns. 2. Position affected extremities out of synergy; place in extension for flexion synergy pattern and place in flexion for extension synergy pattern. 3. Alternate between supine, right and left side-lying, and prone positions.	This is the first step of progressive mobilization and helps prevent the onset of contractures and formation of pressure ulcers. After a stroke, muscle tone is disordered, affecting ability and treatment. Muscle tone is the degree of tension or "readiness" in a muscle at rest, as determined by messages from the brain. (See Table 22.1, page 233.)
Do passive ROM exercises twice a day on affected extremities.	The ROM exercises maintain flexibility of the joints and prevent contractures.
Assist patient to do active range-of-motion (AROM) exercises on unaffected extremities.	The AROM exercises maintain conditioning on the unaffected side so the patient will be able to eventually perform self-ROM exercises independently.

Nursing Interventions	Rationales
Teach patient to do self-ROM exercises as soon as patient is ready.	This is an indication of independence and may further motivate the patient.
Use bridging techniques to assist the patient to move in bed.	As the patient gains strength, independent bed movement will be possible. Self-transfer techniques can be initiated when the patient is able to carry out bed mobility independently.
Gradually increase upright activity by elevating the head of the bed, placing the bed in reverse Trendelenburg position at intervals, or using a tilt table.	This prepares the patient for transfer activities and lowers the risk of orthostatic hypotension.
Assess patient to determine readiness to learn transfer skills and to select appropriate transfer technique. Consider the following: 1. trunk stability 2. weight-bearing ability 3. amount of assistance needed (2 persons or 1 person) 4. ability to understand instructions 5. size of patient 6. ability to come to standing position	Method of transfer is determined by the patient's abilities.
Explain the transfer procedure and tell the patient how to help.	This is the first step to independent transfer.
Place bed in lowest position and lock the wheels. Make sure the patient is wearing well-fitting shoes with nonskid soles.	Implementing safety measures will avoid accidents during transfer.
Avoid placing your hands under the patient's shoulders and never allow the patient's hands to be placed on your body.	Elderly shoulders are frail and can be easily injured. The patient may lose balance or be disoriented and inadvertently grab your neck, causing loss of balance and neck injury.
Place a transfer (gait) belt snugly around patient's waist for standing transfers.	The transfer belt allows the caregiver to assist in transfer without handling the patient's body.

Nursing Interventions	Rationales
Allow the patient to sit on the edge of the bed for a few minutes before standing.	This may avoid orthostatic hypotension.
Support the weak arm during the transfer.	Shoulder subluxation can occur if the affected arm is allowed to hang without support.
Instruct the patient before standing to 1. move forward to the edge of the bed or chair seat. 2. separate the knees for a wide base of support. 3. lean forward and move the feet slightly back. 4. check the feet before standing. 5. support his or her weak leg. 6. use strong hand (both hands if possible) to push off the bed or chair to come to standing position.	This position facilitates rising to a standing position. Supporting the weak leg prevents the leg from sliding out of control. Most people who have had a stroke suffer a loss of proprioception and cannot determine the position of the legs and feet without looking at them. The patient must learn to check the position of the extremities to avoid injuring the affected foot. NOTE: The use of a trapeze may be detrimental for the patient who is attempting to regain mobility skills. This activity strengthens the biceps muscles but does little for the triceps, which are needed for such actions as pushing off of the bed or chair to come to a standing position.
Assess the patient for readiness for ambulation. The patient should be able to 1. sit without back or arm support. 2. stand on both feet without falling. 3. use the unaffected arm to hold and bear down on a walking device. 4. remain upright while ambulating. 5. bear weight in the unaffected leg to compensate for the hemiplegia in the other leg.	Walking is a complex motor act that depends on several other skills before it can be mastered. The patient must be able to carry out all previous mobility techniques competently before learning to walk. An ankle-foot orthosis compensates for weakness but does not improve muscle strength. Consult with the physical therapist for ambulation techniques.

Nursing Interventions	Rationales
Measure the patient for the appropriate assistive device and teach the patient how to use the device with the appropriate gait.	An assistive device provides stability and compensation for the loss of strength in the affected leg.
Put a gait belt on the patient during ambulation: 1. Stand on the affected side and a little behind the patient with your right hand on the gait belt and your left hand in front of the affected shoulder. 2. Assume a wide base of support and coordinate steps.	Standing and moving with the patient on the affected side is not only safer but also helps the patient attend to that side of the body. The gait pattern after a stroke is affected by uneven step lengths, a lack of flexion in the affected hip, and vaulting on the strong side.

► NURSING DIAGNOSIS: *High Risk for Injury*

Risk Factors
- Loss of proprioception
- Unilateral neglect and hemianopsia
- Spatial analysis deficits
- Hemianesthesia

Patient Outcomes
The patient will remain free of injury.

Nursing Interventions	Rationales
Teach the patient to check the position of the affected leg and foot before transfers and ambulation.	The loss of position sense (proprioception) occurs with alteration of the kinesthetic sense. The proprioceptors located in the muscles transfer information used to coordinate muscle activity. The loss of this ability means the patient is not aware of the position of the affected extremities without looking at them. A paralyzed foot often

Nursing Interventions	Rationales
	assumes a position of inversion which can cause injury and falling if the patient attempts to stand.
Assist the patient to maintain body alignment when sitting and standing. Provide guidance in activities that require spatial judgments to avoid injuries.	Spatial deficits are reflected in the inability to judge distance, size, position, rate of movement, form, and relation of parts to wholes. The patient with a spatial analysis deficit lives in a world of tilted space and will slump to the affected side. The patient may bump into door frames or may miss the saucer when setting down a cup. The patient may eventually assimilate compensatory techniques to overcome the deficit.
Arrange the room so the unaffected side is facing the door when in bed or chair. Talk to the patient and present activities from the unaffected side. During meals, arrange the food so it is within the field of vision. Place the call light and other needed objects on the unaffected side. Teach the patient to increase the field of vision by scanning. Give as much feedback as possible about the affected side. Place the affected arm within the line of vision.	Hemianopsia means the patient is blind to objects on the affected side. When unilateral neglect is present, the patient does not attend to the body on the affected side. The reader is advised to investigate the literature to learn the Bobath approach. With this approach, care is planned to help the patient regain awareness of the affected side. The objective is to improve function on the affected side so that the affected side and unaffected side will ultimately function together in harmony.
Check the affected side frequently for signs of injury, pressure ulcers, or infection. Avoid situations that can result in thermal injuries.	Hemianesthesia results in loss of sensation on the affected side.

▶ **NURSING DIAGNOSIS:** *Self-Care Deficits (Grooming, Hygiene, Feeding)*

Related To perceptual deficits due to stroke.

Defining Characteristics
- Agnosia
- Apraxia
- Figure-ground deficit
- Sequencing disorder

Patient Outcomes
The patient will perform the activities of daily living (ADL) with minimal assistance.

Nursing Interventions	Rationales
Label frequently used items with the appropriate names. Tell the patient the names of objects used for ADL. Have the patient feel the object.	Agnosia may be a visual, auditory, or somatosensory deficit in which an individual with normal visual perception does not recognize a common item such as a comb or toothbrush. The stimulus has no meaning or the meaning is distorted. There are several forms of agnosia.
Demonstrate and/or gesture so the patient can imitate the activity. Avoid lengthy instructions. For example, place a bowl of cereal in front of the patient and the spoon in the patient's hand, saying, "This is your spoon and this is your cereal." Use hand-over-hand techniques with eating, grooming, and hygiene procedures.	If apraxia is present, the patient cannot carry out a familiar motor act, despite the absence of paralysis. For example, the patient may know what a comb is but be unable to pick it up and use it appropriately. There are several forms of apraxia. There may be an automatic response if the object is given to the patient with minimal or no verbal instructions using hand-over-hand techniques.
Arrange items on surfaces with contrasting color. Avoid clutter. Place only the items needed in front of the patient.	The patient with figure-ground deficits is unable to distinguish foreground from background.
Lay out items in the order in which they are to be used or put on.	The patient is unable to carry out specific components or steps in a task in the correct order or sequence. This is most often seen with dressing.

▶ NURSING DIAGNOSIS: *Altered Thought Processes*

Related To deficits in attention, concentration, and memory.

Defining Characteristics
- Inability to focus on an activity long enough to initiate or to complete the activity.
- Inability to retain information for later retrieval.

Patient Outcomes
The patient will complete ADL with minimal assistance.

Nursing Interventions	Rationales
Reduce stimulation during periods of instruction.	Any distraction from the environment or other people will decrease the ability to attend to and concentrate on the task being presented.
Provide explicit cues during instruction. These may be verbal, visual, tactile, or demonstrated, depending on the patient's cognitive abilities and perceptual skills.	Cues keep the patient on track and are helpful in counteracting deficits in attention, concentration, and memory.
Use simple, brief instructions and cues. Give one step at a time.	The patient cannot remember lengthy instructions.
Establish environmental cues. Label and keep items in the same place. Provide large-numbered calendars and clocks. Maintain consistency in routines and procedures.	Help the patient remain oriented.

▶ NURSING DIAGNOSIS: *Impaired Verbal Communication*

Related To verbal apraxia, dysarthria, and aphasia due to destruction of brain cells in speech centers of the brain.

Defining Characteristics
- Difficulty expressing thoughts verbally
- Difficulty in comprehending others

Patient Outcomes

The patient will
- experience fewer periods of frustration due to impaired communication.
- develop successful communication techniques.

Nursing Interventions	Rationales
Consult with the physician for an evaluation by a speech pathologist.	The skills and knowledge of the speech pathologist are required for the evaluation and treatment of language and speech disorders.
Implement these general guidelines for communicating with patients with verbal apraxia: 1. Provide a picture notebook of objects that relate to the patient's immediate needs: a toilet, bed, glass of water, etc. The patient can point to the correct object. 2. Provide a magic slate if the patient can write. 3. Provide a notebook of common, frequently used words if the patient can read. 4. If the patient acquires a new word in speech therapy, reinforce the use of the new word. 5. Encourage the use of gestures.	When verbal apraxia (a disorder of speech) is present, the brain is not sending the information to the muscles that enable the patient to produce speech voluntarily. If the apraxia is mild, there may be intelligible speech but inconsistent sound substitutions.
Listen to the patient and concentrate on what is being said. Be sure the environment is quiet: 1. Listen for consistency. 2. Do not simplify your communication. Ask questions that do not require lengthy answers. 3. Ask the patient to think about the movements of the tongue, lips, and cheeks when speaking. 4. Consider a communication board for the patient who is extremely unintelligible.	Dysarthria (a disorder of speech) is due to a weakness or paralysis of one or more of the muscles used in speaking. There may be a combination of disorders characterized by difficulties with phonation, articulation, resonance, and rate and rhythm of speech. Dysarthria does not affect comprehension.

Nursing Interventions	Rationales
Follow the guidelines for communicating with persons with aphasia (see Table 22.2, page 234).	Aphasia (a language impairment) involves all language modalities. It affects speaking, reading, writing, comprehension, object recognition, and arithmetic. All staff can communicate with the patient if consistent guidelines are followed.

▶ **NURSING DIAGNOSIS:** *Impaired Swallowing*

Related To neuromuscular impairment.

Defining Characteristics
- Evidence of difficulty in swallowing through observation and on video-recorded fluoroscopy
- Stasis of food in oral cavity
- Coughing/choking while eating

Patient Outcomes
The patient will swallow without aspiration.

Nursing Interventions	Rationales
Assess for the presence of these criteria before feeding the patient if impaired swallowing is suspected. Patient can 1. adequately respond. 2. control drooling. 3. produce audible cough. 4. voluntarily swallow. 5. exhibit gag reflex when evaluator strokes right and left pharyngeal walls with tongue blade.	To swallow there must be adequate control of oral muscle movement as noted by absence of drooling. The ability to cough and gag minimizes the risk of aspiration.
Consult with physician for swallowing evaluation via video-recorded fluoroscopy by speech pathologist if assessment reveals impaired swallowing.	Video-recorded fluoroscopy is used to make a definitive diagnosis of impaired swallowing.

Nursing Interventions	Rationales
Begin with foods that require very little manipulation when feeding is started: semisolid foods of medium consistency like mashed potatoes, casseroles, scrambled eggs, and custards. Use a commercial thickener with liquids to create the right consistency. Avoid milk, citrus juices, and water in the beginning.	These foods allow the patient to concentrate on swallowing rather than chewing, and less control is required to manipulate them through the oral cavity. Liquids are also difficult to control. Water may present problems because of the minimal sensory stimulation associated with water. Milk, milk products, and citrus juices stimulate the production of saliva. Thickening the liquids does not change the taste and makes them more manageable.
Allow a rest period before eating.	Fatigue increases the risk of aspiration.
Position patient at a 60°–90° angle before, during, and for 1 h after eating, whether in bed or in a chair.	Correct positioning minimizes the risk of aspiration.
Maintain head in midline with the neck slightly flexed during swallowing.	This position facilitates the passage of food through the pharynx.
Face the patient and avoid an impression of haste.	Facing the patient provides opportunity to the feeder to evaluate the eating process. If the feeder appears hurried, the patient may try to eat faster, increasing the risk of aspiration.
Minimize distractions, keep conversation minimal, and do not ask questions until swallowing is completed.	All of the patient's attention has to focus on eating.
Allow the patient to see and smell the food, giving verbal descriptions if necessary. Use a regular metal teaspoon, giving only one-half teaspoonful at a time. Ask the patient to feel the spoon on the lips and then the tongue.	Sensory cues promote awareness of eating.

Nursing Interventions	Rationales
Place the food on the intact side of the mouth. Teach the voluntary swallow by instructing the patient to hold the food in the mouth while thinking about swallowing and then to swallow twice. Look for the rise of the larynx to indicate swallowing is completed.	Buccal pocketing of food in the cheek on the weak side is common with patients who have strokes.
Check for a clear mouth before proceeding.	Minimize risk of aspiration.

▶ **NURSING DIAGNOSIS:** *Situational Low Self-Esteem*

Related To changes in functional abilities resulting from stroke.

Defining Characteristics
- Verbalization of negative feelings about self in regard to loss of abilities
- Difficulty making decisions

Patient Outcomes
The patient will
- verbalize acceptance of self and situation.
- verbalize acceptance of changes in life-style.
- actively strive to utilize strengths.

Nursing Interventions	Rationales
Assess for signs of severe or prolonged grieving.	The patient needs to grieve the loss of the former person. However, signs of severe or prolonged grieving indicate the need for counseling.
Assess patient's interactions with significant other(s).	Other individuals may be reinforcing the concepts of helplessness and invalidism.
Listen in nonjudgmental fashion to patient's comments about situation.	Various aspects of a situation affect each person differently. For example, one person may be acutely distressed by impaired communication but accept

Nursing Interventions	Rationales
	impaired mobility. The patient's concerns may not be verbalized directly, especially those that relate to sexual identity.
Set limits on maladaptive behaviors. Facilitate attempts to identify positive behaviors.	The patient may adapt to the situation more easily when limits are acknowledged.
Continue to assist patient to reach optimal levels of functional performance, stressing abilities. Work with significant other(s) in making necessary adaptations in physical environment to encourage increased independence. Allow to make decisions whenever possible and within the realm of capability. Provide necessary assistance to maximize physical appearance.	Avoid formation of learned helplessness which results from loss of control and which can become a chronic state with feelings of hopelessness and uselessness.

▶ NURSING DIAGNOSIS: *Family Coping, Potential for Growth*

Related To spouse's positive approach to patient's illness.

Defining Characteristics
- Spouse expresses desire to learn about stroke and the problems associated with stroke.
- Spouse seeks information from staff on how to assist patient in ADL.
- Spouse shares affection and attention with patient.

Patient Outcomes
The spouse and patient will
- verbalize willingness and readiness to undertake responsibilities related to recovery of patient.
- verbalize feelings of self-confidence with their abilities and the progress being made.

Nursing Interventions	Rationales
Invite patient and spouse to care-planning conferences.	The patient and spouse are members of the health care team. Communication between the two is enhanced if both are given the opportunity to discuss care, treatment, and progress.
Invite the spouse to observe and learn assistive techniques used by staff for mobility and self-care.	The spouse can begin to participate in care before discharge.
Consult with spouse to 1. discuss what spouse can do to help with care. 2. keep spouse informed of patient's condition and progress. 3. answer questions. 4. help him or her learn to communicate with patient. 5. participate in discharge planning.	The spouse will gain self-confidence in ability to assist patient in recovery and rehabilitation. Making decisions regarding discharge gives the spouse "ownership" in problem resolution.
Provide privacy during spousal visits.	Opportunities for physical closeness, affection, and intimacy can facilitate the relationship toward further growth.
Encourage the spouse to 1. discuss how the illness will affect the family. 2. discuss feelings about the patient's illness. 3. talk about negative feelings. 4. attend support group for family caregivers.	The spouse needs support in order to provide support for the patient. There are many fears, feelings of guilt, anger, and resentment associated with illness of a spouse. Listening to the spouse can provide clues about need for teaching and/or counseling.

DISCHARGE PLANNING/CONTINUITY OF CARE

- Assess current functional abilities for ADL.
- Evaluate availability of significant other(s) to provide assistance with ADL.
- Arrange for further rehabilitation, if necessary, at a rehabilitation hospital or long-term care facility.
- Arrange for home health care if necessary.
- Evaluate physical environment of home setting and make suggestions for adaptations.
- Contact durable medical equipment supplier for needed items such as wheelchair, cane, or hospital bed.

Clinical Clip

- The drug ticlopidine hydrochloride has been approved as a preventive therapy for patients who have had TIAs or recent thrombotic strokes and for use in reducing stroke risk.

- The incidence of stroke peaks in the morning and is associated with physical activity. Advise patients with cardiovascular problems to avoid strenuous exercise and smoking until they have been out of bed for a few hours.

Table 22.1 • Stages of Recovery in CVA

1. Flaccid
2. Spasticity, weak voluntary movement
3. Synergy movement, spasticity
4. Active movement, decreased spasticity
5. Independent movement, minimal spasticity
6. Isolated movement and voluntary control

Spasticity is an increased state of tension in the muscle and is a result of hyperactivity of the stretch reflex. Stretch reflex refers to the muscle contraction that occurs when a pull is exerted upon the tendon of the muscle. Impulses are sent to the spinal cord through sensory nerves. Motor nerves send messages to make the necessary changes in the muscle. In the presence of central nervous system (CNS) damage, the balance between stimuli that increase muscle sensitivity and those that decrease muscle sensitivity is altered. The stretch reflex which is normally inhibited by the CNS becomes overactive. The muscles are more sensitive to stimuli and this causes the formation of synergies. A synergy is an abnormal pattern of movement seen with increased levels of spasticity. The muscles tend to move together; voluntary movement of one joint is not possible. For example, an attempt to move the affected elbow would result in movement of all joints of that arm. There are typical synergy patterns:

1. Flexion synergy pattern of upper extremity
   - Rotation and retraction of scapula
   - Internal rotation and adduction of shoulder
   - Flexion of elbow, wrist, and fingers
2. Extension synergy pattern of upper extremity
   - Rotation and retraction of scapula
   - Internal rotation and adduction of shoulder
   - Extension of elbow
   - Flexion of wrist and fingers

Table 22.1 • *continued*

3. Flexion synergy pattern of lower extremity
   - Retraction of pelvis
   - Flexion and external rotation of hip
   - Flexion of knee and ankle
4. Extension synergy pattern of lower extremity
   - Retraction of pelvis
   - Extension and internal rotation of hip
   - Knee extension
   - Plantar flexion of ankle
   - Eversion of foot

Table 22.2 • Communication Guidelines for Aphasia

Be relaxed and calm. Eliminate environmental distractions and noise when communicating.

Treat the patient as an adult. Intellect is not impaired.

Avoid the temptation to talk louder; impaired hearing is not the problem.

Avoid showing disapproval or shock when the patient swears. The patient may retreat, refusing to attempt speech entirely.

Call the patient by name before attempting communication.

Talk to the patient while giving nursing care.

Speak slowly and distinctly without dragging out the words or overarticulating.

Talk about concrete topics. There may be difficulty comprehending abstract ideas.

Use short, complete phrases, especially if a response is needed or instructions are being given.

Talk in a sequential, organized manner, keeping related topics together.

Check comprehension by asking a question based on a previous statement. Ask questions that require short answers or yes-and-no answers. Comprehension may also be evaluated by watching facial expressions. Check the accuracy of yes-and-no answers by asking a question with a no answer that is within the realm of comprehension: "Are you under 50 years of age?"

Be an active listener. Maintain eye contact, stop the activity for a moment, reflect on the words, and ask questions that flow from the comments. Give the patient time to prepare and deliver the message.

Acknowledge the patient's frustration: "You're having a hard time with that word. Let's talk about something else and then you can try it again later."

Table 22.2 • *continued*

Give opportunities to use automatic speech such as greetings and other social exchanges.

Allow the patient to speak for him/herself. Anticipating comments and voicing them for the patient can impede progress.

Try to maintain consistency in routine, caregivers, and environment.

Allow the patient to make decisions consistent with abilities and encourage to do as much as possible.

Provide appropriate opportunities for socialization.

BIBLIOGRAPHY

Adkins, E. R. H. (1991). Nursing care of clients with impaired communication. *Rehabilitation Nursing, 16*(2), 74–76.

Baker, A. C. (1993). The spouse's positive effect on the stroke patient's recovery. *Rehabilitation Nursing, 18*(1), 30–33.

Bronstein, K. S. (1994). Ticlopidine hydrochloride: Its current use in cerebrovascular disease. *Rehabilitation Nursing, 19*(1), 17–20.

Buelow, J. M., & Jamieson, D. (1990). Potential for altered nutritional status in the stroke patient. *Rehabilitation Nursing, 15*(5), 260–263.

Cole-Arvin, C., Notich, L., & Underhill, A. (1994). Identifying and managing dysphagia. *Nursing 94, 24*(1), 48–49.

Cooke, E. A., & Thigpen, R. (1993). Identification and management of cognitive and perceptual deficits. *Rehabilitation Nursing, 18*(5), 314–317.

Galarneau, L. (1993). An interdisciplinary approach to mobility and safety education for caregivers and stroke patients. *Rehabilitation Nursing, 18*(6), 395–399.

Mitiguy, J. (1991). The brain under attack. *Headlines, 2*(3), 2.

Needham, J. F. (1993). *Gerontological nursing—a restorative approach.* Albany, NY: Delmar.

Ragsdale, D., Yarbrough, S., & Lasher, A. T. (1993). Using social support theory to care for CVA patients. *Rehabilitation Nursing, 18*(3), 154–161, 172.

Rosenthal, S. G., et al. (1993). Perceived needs of wives of stroke patients. *Rehabilitation Nursing, 18*(3), 148–153.

Salter, J., Camp, Y., Pierce, L. L., & Mion, L. C. (1991). Rehabilitation nursing approaches to cerebrovascular accident: A comparison of two approaches. *Rehabilitation Nursing, 16*(2), 62–66.

$\mathcal{H}$UNTINGTON'S DISEASE

Huntington's Disease (HD) is an autosomal dominant disorder of the central nervous system characterized by choreiform movements, cognitive impairments, and psychiatric disorders. Each child of a parent with HD has a 50% chance of inheriting the disease. Both males and females with the Huntington's gene can pass the disease to either sons or daughters. The disease does not "skip" a generation. If a person at risk does not have the gene, any children born to that person will be free of the disease and the chain is broken forever in that branch of the family tree. Persons who carry the gene will develop the disease if they live long enough and they may pass the gene on to the next generation. Although the gene is present at birth, symptoms do not usually appear until ages 35–45. However, symptoms may begin anytime from early childhood until old age. The disease is always progressive and irreversible. Currently, there is no treatment that can cure, delay, or slow the course of the disease. Medications may alleviate manifestations of the disease related to involuntary movements, irritability, and depression. There are no remissions with HD. It may, however, stabilize for long periods of time. The disease may progress rapidly over a few years or slowly over 15–20 years.

ETIOLOGIES
- Huntington's disease gene: People with HD have too many copies of a small section of the HD gene.

CLINICAL MANIFESTATIONS
NOTE: There is not a specific sequence in which the three groups of symptoms appear. The disorder of movement is the major physical clinical manifestation of HD.

Physical
- involuntary movements
  - chorea
  - myoclonus

–dystonia (spasm of the muscles in the shoulders, head, and trunk)
–athetosis (a writhing, involuntary movement of the hands, face, and tongue)
- abnormalities of voluntary movement
  –clumsiness
  –bradykinesia
  –slowing of response time
  –inability to sustain a voluntary movement
- dysrhythmic speech
- dysphagia
- loss of bowel and bladder control

Cognitive
- subcortical dementia
  –lapses of memory
  –impaired judgment

Emotional
- vague
- listless
- apathetic
- indifferent
- easily irritated and quick to anger
- emotional lability
- impulsive behavior
- antisocial behavior and withdrawal from the environment
- misuse of drugs or alcohol
- depression or bipolar depression with manic features
- psychosis with hallucinations and delusions.

CLINICAL/DIAGNOSTIC FINDINGS
Diagnosis is based upon the following:
- family history
- physical examination
- predictive test
- diagnostic tests to rule out other neurological disorders

▶ NURSING DIAGNOSIS: *High Risk for Aspiration*

Risk Factors
- Impaired swallowing
- Involuntary movements of tongue, lips, and cheeks during eating

Patient Outcomes

The patient will
- swallow without aspiration.
- maintain adequate nutritional status.

Nursing Interventions	Rationales
Provide foods that are more easily manipulated in the mouth: thickened liquids and pureed foods with a thicker consistency. Avoid foods with two consistencies, such as vegetable soup, and avoid foods that do not easily form a bolus, such as ground meat.	Eating requires energy and concentration for persons with HD. Simplify the process as much as possible.
Eliminate all environmental stimuli during eating.	Persons with HD are easily distracted, which increases the risk for aspiration.
Position in good body alignment with head slightly tilted forward. Use verbal cues and remind patient to swallow. Feed slowly and have patient remain upright for at least 30 min after eating.	Reduce the risk of aspiration.
Teach all caregivers how to perform the Heimlich maneuver for obstructed airway. Have suction equipment close by.	Prompt action is required for obstructed airway.
Provide a high-calorie, nourishing diet. Monitor daily food intake and weigh weekly.	Persons with HD need twice the normal amount of calories per day because of the constant, involuntary physical activity.

▶ NURSING DIAGNOSIS: *High Risk for Injury*

Risk Factors
- Involuntary movements causing poor coordination and balance
- Poor judgment and impulsivity

Patient Outcomes
The patient will be free of injury.

Nursing Interventions	Rationales
Pad the side rails on the bed.	Prevent abrasions and contusions to extremities.
Provide padded, unrestrictive clothing.	Injury can occur during involuntary movements if clothing is too closely fitted. Padding reduces risk of injury if patient falls.
Provide a bedside commode with padded arms and back.	A commode provides more physical support than a toilet.
Use a wheelchair only for transporting the patient from one place to another. For longer periods of sitting, choose a well-padded chair with adequate head and back support and one that is roomy enough to allow the use of supportive devices to maintain body alignment.	Involuntary movements can cause a wheelchair to tip, causing injury. Extremities can get caught in chairs with open areas.
Avoid the use of restraints.	The use of physical restraints increases the risk of injury.

▶ NURSING DIAGNOSIS: *Impaired Physical Mobility*

Related To unsteady gait due to choreiform movements.

Defining Characteristics
- Shuffling, dancing gait: upper body seems to advance ahead of pelvis and legs
- Inability to walk without assistance
- Difficulty in coming to standing position

Patient Outcomes
The patient will ambulate with assistance two or three times a day.

Nursing Interventions	Rationales
Plan to ambulate when energy levels are highest.	Fatigue further diminishes ambulation skills.
Plan for two persons to assist with ambulation. Apply a gait belt and	Having a person on each side provides counterbalance. Unexpected,

Nursing Interventions	Rationales
have one person on each side of the patient. Walk in a straight corridor, free of clutter and with minimal distractions.	involuntary movements can cause the patient to lunge. Using assistive devices like a cane or walker is not usually safe due to choreic movements of arms.
Teach caregivers how to ease patient to the floor if patient begins to fall.	Trying to prevent the fall can cause injury to caregivers and to the patient.

▶ **NURSING DIAGNOSIS:** *Impaired Verbal Communication*

Related To weakened speech muscles.

Defining Characteristics
• Slurred speech
• Speech volume low and inaudible at times

Patient Outcomes
The patient will be able to communicate needs to staff.

Nursing Interventions	Rationales
Instruct patients to think of a slow start, to take their time, and to talk slowly. Avoid conversation, if possible, when patients are tired.	Trying to talk too fast and talking while fatigued increases difficulty with speaking.
Speak at eye level with patient.	Cues can be picked up by watching patient's mouth.
Ask patient to speak one phrase at a time rather than attempting lengthy sentences. After a phrase is spoken, repeat it after the patient.	This gives an opportunity for a short rest, and the caregiver will know whether or not the patient was understood.
Give verbal or visual feedback when patient is understood. If not understood, ask patient to repeat the phrase with different words.	Different words may be easier to articulate.
Consult with speech pathologist if these interventions are not successful.	Alternative methods of communication may need to be established.

▶ NURSING DIAGNOSIS: *Anticipatory Grieving*

Related To progressive loss of health and dependence.

Defining Characteristics
Verbalization of
- concern that disease will cause great suffering and that family will have to witness this
- distress due to dependency
- guilt feelings in regard to at-risk status of children and grandchildren

Patient Outcomes
The patient will
- feel comfortable expressing feelings honestly.
- maintain control of care as long as desired.
- maintain hope, take one day at a time, and look forward to tomorrow.

Nursing Interventions	Rationales
Actively listen to patient's perceptions, permitting expressions of anger or fear. Be sensitive to and acknowledge patient's feelings. Observe body language and monitor patterns of eating, sleeping, and activity for signs of unexpressed emotions. Respect wishes if patient does not desire to talk.	Recognizing and ventilating feelings facilitates acceptance.
Use touch appropriately if it brings comfort.	Touching can express acceptance of the patient.
Encourage to recall and reminisce about happy moments from the past.	Reminiscing validates the worthiness of the patient's life.
Encourage patient to direct care and to do as much as possible for self. Provide assistance when needed.	The patient can maintain control and can perhaps maintain current levels of mental and physical activity to avoid painful complications.
Avoid giving false reassurance but do not deny hope. Assure that assistance will be given to help deal with each problem as it arises and that everything possible will be done to maintain comfort and dignity.	Everyone needs hope in life. Worrying about tomorrow can expend vast amounts of emotional energy.

Nursing Interventions	Rationales
Use humor therapeutically.	Although the patient's health is deteriorating, it is not natural or tolerable to constantly think of one's impending death. There will be periods of denial; do not push the patient back to reality until the patient is ready.
Discuss with the physician, the patient, and family the patient's wishes in regard to life-extending measures.	The patient has control and the family is relieved of the responsibility of having to make a decision during a time of crisis.

▶ NURSING DIAGNOSIS: *Decisional Conflict (Predictive Testing)*

Related To family members' inability to make a decision regarding predictive testing (see Table 23.1, page 245).

Defining Characteristics
- Verbalization of inability to make decision
- Verbalization of concerns regarding influence of test results on individual family members' futures

Patient Outcomes
Family members will
- verbalize feelings to nurse, physician, social worker, and/or genetic counselor.
- arrive at a decision that is compatible with the desires of the family.
- be supportive of each other regardless of the decision.

Nursing Interventions	Rationales
Provide information to staff regarding predictive testing.	It is not the responsibility of the staff to counsel the family in regard to testing. However, the staff should be well informed so they understand the stress of the family.
Be empathetic to the family, listen, and allow them to verbalize their feelings.	At-risk persons may be "symptom searching"—being on the alert for any indication of HD symptoms. If

Nursing Interventions	Rationales
	this response interferes with their lives, intervention by a mental health professional may be necessary. The spouse of the patient and children's spouses are not at risk. They also have concerns and may become overwhelmed with the uncertainty of their futures. Their concern for the family may cause them to overextend themselves.
Avoid minimizing family concerns, but give realistic hope.	Spouses of at-risk persons may encourage denial. Denial is a necessary coping mechanism, but discounting family concerns increases frustration and anxiety.
Recognize that children of the patient may feel guilty at times.	Guilt may stem from anger toward the parent for "giving" them the disease. This is an expected reaction that must be worked through.
Encourage participation in a support group.	Support groups can provide information and emotional support.

DISCHARGE PLANNING/CONTINUITY OF CARE

If the patient is in a long-term care facility, placement is probably permanent. Measures can be taken to
- provide continuing emotional support of the patient and family.
- provide physical and mental comfort to the patient.

If the patient is at home:
- Help patient arrange for caregiving resources.
- Provide information on predictive testing if family indicates interest.

Clinical Clip

Predictive testing centers are beginning to offer a direct gene test for HD. The test requires blood samples only from the person wishing to be tested and from an affected relative, preferably a parent.

Table 23.1 • Predictive Testing for Huntington's Disease

1. The gene that causes HD has been identified. Treatments and eventually a cure may likely result from this research.
2. The predictive test for HD which became available in 1988 will soon be more accurate.
3. Blood samples are analyzed, and by tracking the inheritance of a marker, predictions can be made of the probability that an at-risk person has inherited the gene.
4. Persons considering testing are required to attend classes and participate in counseling before testing.
5. Psychiatric and psychological screening confirms whether or not there are underlying problems that are beyond the person's power to deal with, given adequate support.
6. Samples from other family members are needed. The exact samples that are required are determined on a case-by-case basis.

BIBLIOGRAPHY

Folstein, S. E. (1989). *Huntington's disease, a disorder of families.* Baltimore, MD: Johns Hopkins University Press.

Huntington's Disease Society of America. (1993). We've got the HD gene, but what does it mean? *The Marker, 6*(2), 4.

Kich, C. R., & Stearns, S. A. (1993). Understanding Huntington's disease: An overview of symptomatology and nursing care. *Geriatric Nursing, 14*(5), 268–271.

National Institute of Neurological Disorders and Stroke. (1992). *Huntington's disease,* Bethesda, MD: National Institutes of Health.

Quaid, K. M. (1991). What to look for in a presymptomatic testing program. *The Marker, 4*(2), 4, 6–7.

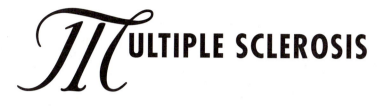

ULTIPLE SCLEROSIS

Multiple sclerosis (MS) is a neurological disease that attacks the myelin sheath, resulting in widely distributed neurological deficits. The myelin sheath is a white, fatty tissue that covers axons and assists in the conduction of nerve impulses. In MS, the ones affected are those that connect neurons in the brain and spinal cord. The disease is not fatal, and death usually results from complications associated with an infectious process or other medical problems. Unpredictability is the key feature of MS. There are four possible courses for the disease (see Table 24.1, page 256). While MS is generally considered a young person's disease, the survival rate is approximately 85% of that for the general population. This means the numbers of older people with MS are steadily increasing.

ETIOLOGIES
- Chemicals produced by the body's T cells and monocytes attack the myelin sheath of nerve cells.

CLINICAL MANIFESTATIONS
- Sensory/motor impairments
  - muscle weakness
  - incoordination
  - ataxia
  - numbness, tingling sensations
  - loss of proprioception
  - Lhermitte's sign (tingling, shocklike sensation that radiates down the trunk and limbs after neck flexion)
  - tremor
- Vision impairments
  - optic neuritis: loss of vision in one eye, blind spots in field of vision, blurring, color blindness
  - diplopia
  - nystagmus (jerky, involuntary eye movements)
- Fatigue
- Communication impairments

CLINICAL/DIAGNOSTIC FINDINGS
- Magnetic resonance imaging (MRI): detects central nervous system (CNS) lesions resulting from MS, found in 90% of persons with clinical diagnosis of MS
- Electrophoresis/cerebrospinal fluid: detects oligoclonal banding, found in 90% of persons diagnosed with MS
- Evoked potentials (EPs): records brain's response to sensory stimuli; slowing of nerve conduction a sign of demyelination

▶ NURSING DIAGNOSIS: *Impaired Physical Mobility*

Related To impaired nerve conduction velocity related to demyelination.

Defining Characteristics
- Spasticity in lower extremities, especially muscles of calf and thigh
- Foot drop and toe dragging during swing phase of gait
- Weakness
- Ataxia

Patient Outcomes
The patient will
- maintain current levels of range of motion.
- increase endurance.
- experience less spasticity.
- improve balance and coordination.
- experience a sense of well-being.

Nursing Interventions	Rationales
Give medication for spasticity as prescribed, about 1 h before exercising. Monitor changes in performance resulting from medication.	Some degree of spasticity may be beneficial if the alternative is weak and rubbery legs. Spasticity may maximize the patient's ability to walk and stand. Drugs eliminating spasticity may unmask weakness that was not previously evident.
Exercise all joints with active range of motion (AROM) twice a day. Do passive range of motion (PROM) or active assistive range of motion (AAROM) if patient is unable to actively exercise. Perform all exercises slowly.	Regular exercising helps prevent stiffness related to spasticity and maintains current levels of range in all joints. Contracture formation and ankylosis may be prevented or delayed. Doing exercises slowly allows joints and muscles to

Nursing Interventions	Rationales
	respond to the stretch by relaxing, avoiding spasticity and clonus.
Perform active resistive exercises if patient's condition permits these exercises: 1. isometric exercises: performed by contracting muscles against resistance but without movement of the joints of the extremities 2. isotonic exercises: joint is moved in the process of contracting the muscles around it NOTE: These exercises should be avoided or used with caution if the patient has compromised cardiovascular function.	Progressive resistive exercise routines strengthen muscles and increase flexibility, thereby improving endurance and coordination. Relaxation after these exercises lasts from 30 min to several hours afterward.
Instruct patient to do repetitive movements of the extremities while lying, sitting, standing, or walking. Consult with physical therapist concerning use of weights during exercises.	Coordination and balance exercises help alleviate ataxia. The weights increase sensory cues.
Advise patient to swim regularly and/or to do stationary cycling if condition permits and opportunity is available. NOTE: Temperature of the water should be under 90 F.	Conditioning of the cardiovascular system is maintained. Swimming in water above this temperature frequently causes extreme weakness in persons with MS.
Teach patient to walk with a wider base of support.	A wide base compensates for disturbances in balance and coordination.
Investigate benefits of ankle-foot orthosis (AFO).	An AFO provides resistance against plantar flexion during the swing phase of the gait. It increases ankle stability when the heel strikes.
Investigate benefits of forearm (Lofstrand) crutches.	Assistive devices can compensate for ataxia and weakness. Forearm crutches allow for use of a four-point gait, which is slow, but which decreases the risk of falling.

Nursing Interventions	Rationales
Consult with physical therapist for evaluation of need for specific gait exercises and walking exercises in a therapeutic pool.	Endurance, balance, and coordination may improve.

▶ NURSING DIAGNOSIS: *Fatigue*

Related To expenditures of energy required to compensate for impaired nerve conduction velocity and consequent attempts to carry out daily activities.

Defining Characteristics
- Frequent complaints of lack of energy
- Patient reports feeling completely weak and drained
- Inability to complete activities due to fatigue

Patient Outcomes
The patient will effectively manage fatigue, as evidenced by participating in activities of choice.

Nursing Interventions	Rationales
Assure that the fatigue is real and due to physical manifestations of the disease. Advise to accept the fatigue instead of trying to fight or deny it.	Patients (and families) often think the fatigue is an emotional problem that the patient can overcome by struggling against it. This increases the fatigue and frustration.
Ask the patient to determine if there is a pattern to the onset of fatigue at particular times during the day.	If a pattern exists, rest periods can be scheduled for these times and activities can be avoided.
Advise the patient to establish priorities for the activities that are personally most important.	Available energy can be utilized for activities that must be done (activities of daily living and exercise) and for those that provide enjoyment and increase the quality of life. For example, if the patient wishes to attend an evening party, other nonessential activities can be

Nursing Interventions	Rationales
	withheld during the day, allowing for additional rest time.
Advise to avoid situations that expose the patient to heat: 1. take cool showers, baths 2. install an air conditioner and/or fans and dehumidifier for hot, summer days 3. ride in air conditioned cars 4. dress in light clothing 5. eat and drink cool foods and beverages 6. reduce fevers promptly 7. swim in pools with temperatures below 90 F.	Persons with MS are often heat sensitive. Problems associated with fatigue, gait, and muscle weakness are intensified to the point where any activity is futile.
Encourage the use of assistive devices such as a walker, a quad cane, forearm (Lofstrand) crutches, or a wheelchair on days when fatigue is worse or when more energy is required to complete specific tasks.	The manifestations of MS are very erratic, often changing from day to day. The patient should not be encouraged to prematurely acquiesce to assistive devices, but should be guided to a realistic acceptance of fluctuating abilities.

▶ **NURSING DIAGNOSIS:** *Impaired Verbal Communication (Dysarthria)*

Related To neurological involvement of speech musculature.

Defining Characteristics
A combination of disorders characterized by difficulties with the following:
- phonation
- articulation
- resonance
- rate and rhythm of speech
- associated problems with swallowing (difficulty controlling saliva) and/or breathing

Patient Outcomes
The patient will
- experience fewer periods of frustration due to impaired communication.
- develop techniques for successful communication.

Nursing Interventions	Rationales
Consult with a speech pathologist in regard to a swallowing evaluation. Monitor for signs of aspiration.	Patients with dysarthria frequently have concurrent dysphagia as a result of weakness of the muscles used for both speech and swallowing. This increases the risk of aspiration.
Listen carefully and concentrate on what is being said. Be sure the environment is quiet.	The problem is often one of volume; muscle weakness precludes the ability to speak louder.
Listen for consistency in errors of sound.	Impaired articulation may produce sounds that are in error, but if they are consistent, caregivers can interpret what is being said.
Ask questions that do not require lengthy answers.	Since the underlying problem is one of muscle weakness, the patient may be able to speak for short periods but will be more difficult to understand as fatigue becomes greater.
Avoid simplifying speech. Talk to the patient in an adult manner.	Dysarthria does not affect comprehension or intelligence.
Ask the patient to think about the movements of the tongue, lips, and cheeks when speaking.	Concentrating on the acts required for speaking may enable the patient to assume more control over the speech muscles.
Teach the patient to slow the rate of speech.	More time is available for the tongue to compensate for the loss of control.
Consult with the speech pathologist to investigate the following: 1. the benefits of speech therapy 2. exercises for specific speech muscles 3. alternate modes of communication	All efforts should be made to facilitate communication. Being able to communicate successfully enhances socialization and decreases the frustration of the patient and caregivers.

▶ NURSING DIAGNOSIS: *Reflex Incontinence*

Related To weakness of the detrusor muscle and spasticity of the sphincter due to disease involvement of the third and fourth sacral nerves.

Defining Characteristics
- Urinary hesitancy
- Sensation of incomplete bladder emptying after voiding

Patient Outcomes
The patient will
- have decreased postvoid residuals (PVR).
- remain free of urinary tract infections.

Nursing Interventions	Rationales
Complete a bladder management assessment (see Urinary Incontinence, page 175).	Assessment data provide direction for intervention.
Instruct the patient to establish a regular voiding schedule. Teach methods to ensure bladder emptying: 1. Tap the suprapubic area. 2. Stroke the glans penis (males). 3. Rub the thighs. 4. Gently pull the pubic hair. 5. Gently touch the urinary meatus with toilet tissue.	These actions trigger detrusor contractions.
Encourage intake of three or four glasses of cranberry juice a day. Maintain a minimum daily fluid intake of 2,500 mL. Consult with physician on benefits of taking vitamin C daily.	Cranberry juice and vitamin C acidify the urine. Citrus juices tend to increase urinary pH. Maintaining urinary pH <6 and adequate fluid intake reduce the risks of urinary tract infection.
Measure PVR by catheterization or bedside pelvic ultrasound.	A PVR >100–200 mL increases the risk of bladder infection.
Consult with physician regarding benefits of urinary antiseptics for a significant PVR.	Urinary antiseptics reduce the incidence of infection by generating formaldehyde salts in the urine.
Consider intermittent catheterization for consistently high PVR. Teach the patient to do clean self-catheterization if there is adequate dexterity in arms and fingers.	Symptoms are relieved and frequency of urinary tract infections are reduced.

▶ NURSING DIAGNOSIS: *Constipation*

Related To disease involvement of third and fourth sacral nerves.

Defining Characteristics
- Inability to defecate
- Hard-formed stools

Patient Outcomes
The patient will have regular soft-formed bowel movements.

Nursing Interventions	Rationales
Establish daily routine: 1. minimum daily fluid intake of 2,500 mL 2. diet including high-fiber foods 3. regular toileting schedule according to patient's former habits, allowing privacy, physical comfort, and adequate time 4. consistent exercise routine in accordance with patient's abilities	These measures promote regular bowel evacuation.
Administer psyllium or docusate sodium if needed. Give adequate fluids with both medications to ensure effectiveness.	Psyllium forms a bulky gel in the intestines, stimulating peristalsis. Docusate sodium helps water penetrate and soften hard, dry stools, easing passage of stool through the colon.

▶ NURSING DIAGNOSIS: *High Risk for Impaired Skin Integrity*

Risk Factors
- Immobility
- Decreased sensation

(See Pressure Ulcer, page 9.)

▶ NURSING DIAGNOSIS: *Altered Family Processes*

Related To long-term illness of the patient and the role changes experienced by both partners.

Defining Characteristics
- Inability of partners to communicate feelings to each other
- Family uninvolved in activities outside of the household
- Expressed negative feelings of both partners about the situation

Patient Outcomes
The patient and spouse will
- express their feelings openly and constructively.
- establish a routine that is agreeable to both of them.
- utilize effective problem-solving skills.
- express understanding of MS and its effects.
- enjoy a relationship that is satisfying to both partners.

Nursing Interventions	Rationales
Encourage the patient and spouse to communicate with each other openly, honestly, and constructively. Refer to counseling if necessary.	Long-term chronic illness takes a toll on relationships. When one is sick, two need help. Older persons who have MS have generally had it for several years. Patterns have been established that may not be conducive to mutual understanding.
Refer spouse and patient to MS support group.	Persons who were diagnosed with MS several years ago were often not provided with information concerning the disease and its effects. Issues of a caregiver are different from the issues faced by the patient. Both people need support and understanding.
Evaluate the abilities of the patient to assume some of the household abilities. Discuss with both partners an amicable arrangement that will increase the self-esteem of the patient and relieve the spouse of some responsibilities.	Incorrect perceptions of the patient and the illness may be formed over the years. The patient may have been placed in a dependent role prematurely and unnecessarily. The spouse assumes more and more responsibilities over the years, becoming fatigued and resentful.
Encourage the couple to reestablish a social life that is agreeable to them both. Advise them to plan the patient's day accordingly so there is energy to enjoy an evening out.	Socialization can add zest and stimulation to the daily routine.

Nursing Interventions	Rationales
Advise the couple that counseling is available for matters concerning sexuality.	When a couple experiences a chronic illness for many years, the healthy partner may view self as a caregiver and lose sight of the sexual aspect of the relationship. Multiple sclerosis has a direct effect on the physiology of sexual response that may begin even in the early stages of the disease. Over the years, the sexual relationship may erode, leaving the needs of both people unmet.

DISCHARGE PLANNING/CONTINUITY OF CARE

For the hospitalized patient returning home:
- Evaluate the ability of the patient and/or family to meet the needs of the patient as described in this chapter.
- Arrange for home health care as indicated by the evaluation.
- Arrange for a homemaker to periodically relieve the spouse.
- Suggest joining a MS support group in the community.

--- Clinical Clip ---

Interferon beta-1b has been approved for use in exacerbating-remitting forms of MS. The product is a protein produced by recombinant deoxyribonucleic acid (DNA) technology and is prescribed to decrease the frequency of recurrent attacks of neurologic dysfunction.

Table 24.1 • Course of Multiple Sclerosis

Benign: mild attacks occurring intermittently with long symptom-free periods

Exacerbating-remitting: periods of illness occurring with acute onset, followed with partial or complete recovery and a plateau of stable disability

Chronic-progressive: a slow, steady course of deterioration with increasing levels of disability

Chronic-relapsing: a continual deterioration with fewer remissions over a period of time

BIBLIOGRAPHY

Chipps, E., Clanin, N., & Campbell, V. (1992). *Neurologic disorders,* St. Louis, MO: Mosby Year-Book.

Frames, R. (1989). Getting a grip on gait. *Inside MS, 7*(1), 27–29.

Kirsch, B. (1993). Too darn hot! *Inside MS, 11*(1), 10–12.

McCann, J. A. S. (1991). *Diagnostic test implications.* Springhouse, PA: Springhouse Corporation.

National Institute of Neurological Disorders and Stroke. (1990). *Multiple sclerosis.* Bethesda, MD: National Institutes of Health.

Shaw, P. (1989). Digging for clues to fatigue. *Inside MS, 7*(4), 16–17.

$\mathscr{P}$ARKINSON'S DISEASE

Parkinson's disease (PD) is a chronic, progressive disorder of the brain, resulting from damage to the extrapyramidal system. The substantia nigra in the cerebrum consists of pigmented cells containing neuromelanin, which produces and stores the neurotransmitter dopamine, which has an inhibitory effect on movement. These cells synapse with the cells in the striatum that control movement, balance, and walking. Messages pass between cells in the substantia nigra and the striatum through dopamine.

ETIOLOGIES
- A deficiency in dopamine production, disturbing the balance between dopamine and acetyl choline

CLINICAL MANIFESTATIONS

Primary
- resting tremor
- rigidity (cogwheeling)
- bradykinesia

Secondary
- fatigue
- dysarthria
- dysphagia
- depression
- dementia

CLINICAL/DIAGNOSTIC FINDINGS
Diagnosis confirmed by assessment of clinical manifestations through
- physical examination
- history

▶ NURSING DIAGNOSIS: *Impaired Physical Mobility*

Related To
- Bradykinesia
- Gait deviations
- Decreased strength
- Endurance

Defining Characteristics
- Shuffling, accelerating gait
- Tendency to stoop forward
- Walking on the balls of the feet
- Lack of arm swing during walking
- Freezing periods: unable to raise either foot from the floor
- Difficulty arising from sitting position

Patient Outcomes
The patient will
- maintain current range of motion (ROM) in all extremities.
- get out of bed independently.
- sit down and arise from the chair independently.
- experience fewer freezing episodes and know what to do when one occurs.
- improve endurance by gradually increasing walking distance.

Nursing Interventions	Rationales
Instruct patient to do 1. ROM exercises twice a day. 2. active ROM with the head and neck and active assistive ROM with other joints in conjunction with stretching. 3. pulley exercises for the shoulders: Install a rope and pulley in a doorway. Sit in a chair underneath and hold one end of the rope in each hand, pulling first with one hand and then the other, fully elevating each hand.	Daily exercises of all joints maintains flexibility, preventing contractures.
Teach to get out of bed by clasping hands either behind the head or in front, rolling body back and forth. Roll onto side and slide feet to edge of bed. Use hands to push to sitting position.	Rolling back and forth increases momentum. Feet will automatically swing to floor.

Nursing Interventions	Rationales
Provide a straight chair with arm rests. Place 2 × 4-in. blocks under back legs. Teach the patient to 1. get out of chair by sliding to the edge with feet about 8 in. apart. 2. place one foot further forward. 3. put weight on the ball of the foot in back and then rock forward and back. 4. on the count of 3, push down with hands on armrests and stand. 5. sit and then back up so chair touches back of legs. 6. bend knees, lean slightly forward, grasp armrests, and slowly lower into chair.	Movement in and out of a chair is facilitated if the front of the chair is lower than the back. Spreading the feet apart with one foot forward broadens the base of support. Rocking increases momentum. Pushing down on armrests utilizes the arm muscles to push the body upright.
Teach patient to improve gait: 1. Wear shoes with a nonstick sole. 2. Use a wide-based gait, keeping feet about 8 in. apart. 3. Think about moving arms in normal swing. 4. Turn corners by keeping feet apart and head up and walking into turn by making a semicircle. 5. Practice marching and walking sideways, backwards, and in circles.	Rubber soles increase the tendency to walk with small, shuffling steps, causing the upper body to lean forward and increasing the risk of falling. A wide gait increases the base of support and minimizes freezing episodes. Arm swing is a part of normal gait. The patient needs to concentrate on the act of walking.
Teach patient to handle freezing episodes: 1. Raise head and relax back on heels without trying to take any more steps. 2. Straighten knees, hips, and trunk. 3. Rock from side to side and then take some marching steps in place. 4. Begin walking by placing heels down first.	Concentration, upright position, and rocking break the freezing action. Beginning with heel strike facilitates normal gait.

▶ NURSING DIAGNOSIS: *Self-Care Deficit (Dressing)*

Related To
- Rigidity of hand
- Tremors
- Tendency to fatigue

Defining Characteristics
- Difficulty with fine motor tasks: manipulating buttons, zippers, snaps, and shoe laces
- Prolonged length of time for dressing

Patient Outcomes
The patient will
- maintain current levels of hand and finger dexterity by carrying out exercises as instructed.
- dress and undress independently, allowing caregiver to help if necessary, preventing fatigue and frustration.

Nursing Interventions	Rationales
Suggest exercises for hands and fingers: 1. Squeeze and mold physical therapy putty with each hand. Use thumbs and index fingers to pinch off small bits. (Putty comes in different consistencies.) 2. Use a hand gripper several times a day. 3. Use thumb and index finger to pick up various sized coins on a table top. 4. Play checkers, put puzzles together.	These exercises strengthen the hands and fingers to help maintain/increase functional skills. Coordination is increased and opposition (thumb-to-finger movement) is improved.
Select loose-fitting and stretchy clothing. Resew buttons on cardigan-style clothing with elastic thread. Replace neckties with clip-on ties. Wear beltless pants/skirts or put belt in garment before dressing. Wear well-fitting slip-on shoes or shoes with elastic laces or velcro closures.	The right type of clothing facilitates dressing and reduces the need for fine motor movements.

Nursing Interventions	Rationales
Help/teach patient to dress: 1. Dress while sitting in a chair. 2. Put on upper body clothing first, putting arms into sleeves, then slipping head into neck opening. 3. Put on socks. 4. Put on pants/skirt next, pulling them up as far as possible while seated; then put on shoes with elastic shoelaces or velcro closures. Use a long-handled shoehorn. 5. Stand up, pull pants/skirt up over hips. Buckle belt first and then close zipper.	This procedure 1. conserves energy, reducing fatigue. 2. facilitates ease in dressing. 3. prevents toes from getting caught in clothing by putting on socks first. 4. eliminates the need to bend forward, reducing the risk of losing balance.

▶ **NURSING DIAGNOSIS:** *Altered Nutrition—Less Than Body Requirements*

Related To difficulty chewing and swallowing and fatigue due to length of time required for eating.

Defining Characteristics
- Inability to finish a meal
- Weight loss
- Complaints of food getting stuck in throat

Patient Outcomes
The patient will
- consume 80–90% of meals without becoming fatigued.
- have fewer episodes of food getting stuck in throat.
- gain ½ lb per week until usual body weight is attained.

Nursing Interventions	Rationales
Consult with speech pathologist or occupational therapist for swallowing evaluation.	Direction can be provided concerning interventions.
Serve six small meals a day, rather than three larger ones.	This may prevent fatigue, enabling patient to consume more food.

Nursing Interventions	Rationales
Serve appetizing, attractive foods that are easy to chew and swallow, rather than pureed foods. Use a commercial thickener for liquids.	Pureed foods are boring and unappetizing. Thickening liquids eases swallowing and reduces the risk of aspiration without altering the taste.
Utilize adaptive devices: 1. thermal plate 2. nonslip mat under plate 3. plate guard 4. stationary flexible straw 5. utensils with built-up handles	These devices will maintain foods at proper temperatures, making them more appetizing, and will allow the patient to maintain independence in eating in an orderly manner.
Position for eating: 1. Maintain body alignment in upright position with hips, knees, and ankles at 90° angles and feet flat on floor. 2. Remain in this position for 30 min after eating. 3. Instruct to take small bites and, after chewing, move food to back of mouth. Tilt head slightly forward before swallowing.	These techniques facilitate swallowing and reduce the risk of aspiration.
Weigh weekly.	Prompt interventions can be implemented if weight loss occurs.
Teach caregiver(s) procedure for obstructed airway.	Prompt action can be taken if aspiration occurs.

▶ NURSING DIAGNOSIS: *Impaired Verbal Communication (Dysarthria)*

Related To
- Rigid vocal muscles
- Stiff mouth
- Stiff facial muscles

Defining Characteristics
- Indistinct speech, accelerating at end of sentences
- Breathy and tremulous voice with decreased volume
- Others have difficulty understanding

Patient Outcomes

The patient will
- attempt to prevent further deterioration of verbal communication by carrying out oral exercises regularly.
- communicate verbally in an understandable manner.

Nursing Interventions	Rationales
Consult with speech pathologist for evaluation. If this is not possible, teach/assist with oral exercises:	Increase flexibility of tongue, mouth, and cheek muscles to improve articulation of speech.

1. Use a mirror to help to do exercises. Practice two to three times a day for 5–10 min. Try them all.
2. Open and close mouth slowly several times. Be sure lips are all the way closed. Pucker lips as for a kiss, hold, then relax. Repeat several times.
3. Spread lips into a big smile, hold, then relax. Repeat several times.
4. Pucker, hold, smile, hold. Repeat this alternative movement several times. Open mouth, then try to pucker with mouth wide open.
5. Close lips tightly and press together. Relax and repeat.
6. Close lips firmly. Slurp all the saliva onto the top of tongue.
7. Open mouth and stick out tongue. Be sure tongue comes straight out of mouth and does not go off to the side. Hold tongue out and then relax and repeat several times. Work toward sticking tongue out farther each day.
8. Stick tongue out and move it slowly from corner to corner of lips. Hold in each corner. Relax and repeat several times. Be sure tongue actually touches the corner each time.

Nursing Interventions

Rationales

9. Stick out tongue and try to reach chin with the tongue tip. Hold it out at the farthest point. Relax, repeat.

10. Stick out tongue and try to reach nose with tongue tip. Pretend to be licking a popsicle from top lip. Hold tongue up as far as possible. Relax, repeat.

11. Stick out tongue. Hold spoon against tip of tongue and try to push spoon even farther away with tongue while hand is holding the spoon readily in place. Hold spoon upright. Repeat pretending to lick a popsicle. Relax. Repeat again.

12. Stick tongue out and pull it back. Repeat as many times and quickly as possible. Relax. Repeat.

13. Move tongue from corner to corner as quickly as possible. Relax. Repeat.

14. Move tongue all around lips in a circle as quickly and as completely as possible. Touch all of upper lip, corner, lower lip, and corner. Relax. Repeat.

15. Open and close mouth as quickly as possible. Be sure lips close each time. Relax. Repeat.

16. Say MA-MA-MA-MA as quickly as possible without losing MA sound. Be sure there is an M sound and an AH sound each time. Relax. Repeat.

17. Say LA-LA-LA-LA as quickly and accurately as possible. Relax. Repeat.

(Source: From *Exercises for the Parkinson Patient with Hints for Daily Living* by Coddington,

Nursing Interventions	Rationales
New York: Parkinson's Disease Foundation. Reprinted by permission.)	
During conversations:	Dysarthric speech is soft and diffi-cult to hear. Fatigue increases the dysarthria. Utilizing air from the lungs for speech and concentrating on speech improve articulation.
1. Limit distractions.	
2. Turn off television or radio.	
3. Provide a quiet, private environ-ment without interruptions.	
4. Face the patient while he or she is talking.	
5. Monitor fatigue level and avoid conversation when tired, asking only yes or no questions if necessary.	
6. Instruct to take in air before speaking and then to speak during exhalation.	
7. Teach to think of lips, tongue, and jaws while concentrating on forming one word at a time.	

▶ NURSING DIAGNOSIS: *High Risk for Infection*

Risk Factors
- Impaired throat and chest movements
- Dysphagia, increasing the risk of aspiration and subsequent pneumonia

Patient Outcomes
The patient will remain free of respiratory tract infections.

Nursing Interventions	Rationales
Advise patient to	Prevent respiratory tract infections.
1. get an influenza immunization each fall and pneumococcal vac-cine if not previously vaccinated.	
2. do breathing exercises to increase chest expansion and lung ventilation (see Chronic	

Nursing Interventions

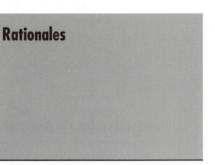

Obstructive Pulmonary Disease,
page 114).
3. maintain adequate fluid intake.
4. avoid exposure to respiratory
infection by avoiding crowds
during peak infection times.

▶ NURSING DIAGNOSIS: *Body Image Disturbance*

Related To visible evidence of disease process and loss of functional abilities.

Defining Characteristics
• Negative comments regarding change in physical condition
• Reluctance to socialize

Patient Outcomes
The patient will
• verbalize positive statements about self and abilities.
• make decisions regarding personal care and activities.
• maintain role in the family by participating in discussions.
• participate in social activities of choice.

Nursing Interventions	Rationales
Encourage patient to direct care by giving choices in activities of daily living, social activities, and scheduling the day.	The patient needs to feel in control of his or her life.
Instruct staff to give the patient opportunity to do as much as possible for self and to intervene with help only when necessary.	Caregivers can avoid promoting the formation of learned helplessness.
Advise family to avoid oversheltering by including patient in all activities and decisions.	Families may feel they are protecting the patient by making plans and decisions without the patient's input.
Encourage family to plan social outings with patient. Plan for early arrival or less busy times.	Socializing in public increases self-confidence. Avoiding crowds minimizes stress.

DISCHARGE PLANNING/CONTINUITY OF CARE

Instruct family to prepare for discharge to home:

- Remove loose rugs and doorsills.
- Arrange space for ambulating around rooms and halls.
- Place lamps and other objects in areas where they will not be accidentally toppled.
- If climbing stairs cannot be avoided, install secure rails on both sides. If disease progresses, an electric chair lift will increase safety and reduce fatigue.
- Install metal or wooden handles on walls adjacent to doorknobs so client can hold handle on wall with one hand while pulling doorknob with the other hand.
- Install elevated toilet seat and bar for support at side of toilet.
- If there is no shower, install hand-held shower device for use in tub. Place nonslip mats on tub floor. Use tub chair.
- Place grab rail on wall next to tub.
- Designate a special chair for client and attach 2×4-in. blocks under back legs or lengthen back legs by 2 in.
- Tie a sheet to the bed post and make a knot in the other end to facilitate getting out of bed.
- Maintain temperature warm enough so client can wear fewer items of clothing. This makes dressing easier.

── Clinical Clip ──

Many patients with PD have restless legs syndrome (crawling sensations in the legs in the evening and during the night). Getting up and walking about can eliminate these unpleasant sensations.

BIBLIOGRAPHY

Chipps, E., Clanin, N., & Campbell, V. (1992). *Neurologic disorders.* St. Louis, MO: Mosby Year-Book.

Coddington, J. (no date). In L. Côté & G. Riedel (Eds.). *Exercises for the Parkinson patient with hints for daily living.* New York: Parkinson's Disease Foundation.

Côté, L., & Riedel, G. (no date). *Exercises for the Parkinson patient with hints for daily living.* New York: Parkinson's Disease Foundation.

DeLaney, J. (1988). *Parkinson's/Alzheimer's disease. Extended care facilities special clinical topics.* Kansas City: Marion Laboratories.

Lieberman, A. N., Gopinathan, G., Neophytides, A., & Goldstein, M. (no date). *Parkinson's disease handbook.* New York: American Parkinson Disease Association.

Talotta, D., & Lisanti, P. (1989). Countering Parkinson's assault on your patient's will. *RN, November, 52*(11), 34–39.

Sensory Conditions

$\mathscr{H}$EARING IMPAIRMENT

$\mathbf{P}$resbycusis is a cause of impaired hearing that is characterized by progressive degeneration of the auditory functions. It includes many types of auditory deterioration. D. A. Ramsdell identified three levels of hearing: primitive, signal, and social. The primitive level includes environmental sounds that facilitate interaction with the world; the sounds of nature, traffic noises, and voices are ways of connecting with the surrounding environment. Warning sounds are at the signal level and include sirens, fire alarms, a baby's cry, calls for help, and car horns. The social level is used for conversational exchange. There are four types of hearing loss: conductive, sensorineural, mixed (a combination of conductive and sensorineural), and central.

ETIOLOGIES
- Conductive: injury, disease, or obstruction that causes a disruption of the conductive mechanism in the outer or middle ear
- Sensorineural: prenatal damage, exposure to excessive noise, ototoxic drugs, normal aging, disease, or injury damage to either the hair cells in the inner ear or the auditory nerve
- Mixed hearing loss: severe infection that damages both the middle and inner ear
- Central hearing loss: damage to the auditory nerve or portion of the brain that recognizes and interprets sounds (a neurological deficit rather than a problem with the ear's ability to receive and transmit sound)

CLINICAL MANIFESTATIONS
- General
  - imprecise speaking patterns if hearing has been impaired for some time
  - sense of isolation
  - depression
  - frustration
- Conductive hearing loss: sounds are not loud enough because sound waves are obstructed
- Sensorineural hearing loss

–affects ability to detect and distinguish high-frequency speech sounds and environmental sounds

–recruitment: the inner ear distorts the sound, telling the brain that it is louder than it really is

–tinnitus: sensation of buzzing or ringing in the ear

• Mixed hearing loss: any of the manifestations listed above
• Central hearing loss: speech/environmental sounds may not be recognized

CLINICAL/DIAGNOSTIC FINDINGS

• Air conduction test determines the degree of loss.
• Bone conduction test and impedance audiometry diagnoses the type of loss.
• Speech reception threshold audiometry determines how loud speech must be in order to be heard.
• Speech discrimination test evaluates how well speech is understood once it is loud enough to hear.

▶ NURSING DIAGNOSIS: *Sensory/Perceptual Alterations/Auditory*

Related To disease, injury, obstruction, or damage to the auditory function.

Defining Characteristics

• Altered abstraction and conceptualization
• Change in behavior
• Apathy
• Change in usual response to auditory stimuli
• Balance problems

Patient Outcomes

The patient will
• receive information regarding hearing loss.
• make decision regarding aural rehabilitation.

Nursing Interventions	Rationales
Assess for ear pain, drainage, inflammation, abnormalities, surgeries, perforations, or impacted cerumen.	Hearing impairment may be temporary and reversible if prompt treatment for the cause is instituted.
Irrigate for cerumen removal if impaction is present and all other findings are negative. If other manifestations are noted, refer to otologist or otolaryngologist.	The elderly undergo changes in the ear which interfere with the normal movement of cerumen to the external ear.

Nursing Interventions	**Rationales**
Evaluate medication regime if above findings are negative.	Many routine medications have potential ototoxic side effects. Tinnitus and sensorineural hearing loss are clinical manifestations of ototoxicity. Elderly persons and those with a history of hearing loss are at risk for ototoxic side effects.
Assess for ototoxicity if medication history reveals the risk for ototoxicity: 1. Ask about symptoms of tinnitus: ringing, roaring, and buzzing noises in ear. 2. Check hearing level with ticking clock. 3. Observe balance and coordination. 4. Observe for loss of proprioception.	If findings indicate ototoxicity, the physician may discontinue medication, reduce the dose, or substitute a medication with less risk.
Arrange for further evaluation of hearing loss.	An otologist can diagnose and treat the physical causes of the loss. The audiologist identifies the degree and type of loss and can prescribe an aural rehabilitation program.
Communicate with audiologist regarding treatment of hearing loss. If a hearing aid is prescribed, instruct patient and other caregivers: 1. Before inserting a hearing aid, check the battery. Each type of aid requires a specific type of battery, and these are not interchangeable. To check, turn the control to "M" or "on." 2. Some models have a "T." This is a telephone switch which activates a telecoil. Telecoil circuitry is built into some hearing aids to facilitate hearing over the telephone. The telephone must be compatible with the telecoil circuitry in order to work. 3. After turning the hearing aid on, test the battery by cupping	The use of hearing aids by older adults is common. These devices require appropriate care to function properly. Patients with impaired vision and limited manual dexterity may require assistance.

Nursing Interventions

your hand over the battery enclosure. A constant whistle indicates a functioning battery. If there is no whistle, replace the battery. Match the positive markings on the battery and battery case.

4. Turn the aid off and the volume down. Place the earmold in the external ear canal, turn it on, and adjust the volume. The hearing aid should fit snugly but comfortably, flush with the ear. The upper extension fits into the upper earlobe.

5. To adjust the volume, talk to the person as you increase the volume. Stop when the person can hear you.

6. If the aid is making squealing noises, check the earmold for placement and fit. Examine the plastic tubing on a behind-the-ear (BTE) aid for cracking or splitting. Test the volume, and if it is too high, turn it down until the squealing stops.

7. If the hearing aid does not work, replace the battery. Check the battery terminals for correct position. If there is corrosion on the battery compartment, remove it with a pencil eraser.

8. Examine the earmold for wax. To remove wax, wash the earmold in warm, soapy water and rinse. Make sure the switch is set on "M" and not on "T." If the sound on a body-type aid clicks on and off, check the wire between the receiver and hearing aid; listen to the hearing aid through the receiver and wiggle the wire. If it is broken or

Nursing Interventions

cracked, the sound will go on and off.

9. If these techniques are not effective, consult the audiologist for repair, replacement, or suggestions.

10. Check the hearing aid daily. Keep a supply of extra batteries on hand and a spare cord for body aids.

11. Keep the aid dry and avoid exposure to temperature extremes. If the aid becomes wet, remove the battery and drain the water. Place the aid in a plastic bag with silica gel to absorb excess moisture.

12. Do not use solvents or lubricants on the hearing aid. Turn the aid off before removing it. Open the battery door to help dry any body moisture that seeps in. Store the aid in its case. Avoid hairspray because it can clog the aid, causing excessive damage.

13. To wash the earmold, detach it from the battery compartment and use warm, soapy water. Rinse with clear water and let it dry before reconnecting. Use a pipe cleaner for the plastic connecting tube.

Rationales

▶ **NURSING DIAGNOSIS:** *Impaired Social Interaction*

Related To inability to hear and understand others.

Defining Characteristics
- Verbalized or observed discomfort in social situations
- Observed use of unsuccessful social interaction behaviors
- Withdrawal due to fear of inability to converse intelligently

Patient Outcome

The patient will verbalize enjoyment of socializing with others.

Nursing Interventions	Rationales
Discuss with patient how aging affects hearing and how hearing loss, in turn, affects communication.	Increase self-image.
Instruct caregivers and family about the problems associated with hearing loss and how they can assist in the communication and socialization process:	The patient's socialization can be enhanced if caregivers and other persons follow these guidelines.

1. Assess hearing and note whether hearing aid is in place if the patient appears inattentive, confused, or slow.
2. Place yourself in good light. Face the patient and light. The patient may read your lips or watch your facial expression.
3. Address patient directly; do not turn your face and do not cover your mouth with your hand. Avoid talking with food or gum in your mouth. Use eye contact.
4. Eliminate distracting noises in the environment and turn off the TV. Lower the tone of your voice. It is easier to hear.
5. Let the patient see you first, then touch the patient's hand or shoulder and call by name. Start with a key word or phrase. Repeat the same words if necessary.
6. Ask a hearing-impaired person if one ear is a "good" ear. If so, stand or sit on that side.
7. Talk at a moderate rate and wait for a response. Speak clearly and distinctly without overarticulating. Keep your voice at the same volume throughout the conversation.

Nursing Interventions

8. Avoid complex, lengthy sentences. Ask only one question at a time. Too many may be difficult to sort out and follow.
9. When changing to a new subject, slow your rate down and make sure the patient is following the change before proceeding. Watch the patient's face for understanding. The patient may pretend to understand, but the face and eyes may indicate puzzlement.
10. Use multiple clues. Point while you are giving instructions.
11. Provide clues as to where sounds are coming from. Intercoms, fire alarms, and other environmental noises may be confusing and frightening.
12. When a hearing-impaired person joins the group, be sure the person knows the subject under discussion. Avoid whispering or carrying on a private discussion with someone else.
13. Do not exclude the patient from "listening" activities. Many hearing-impaired persons can feel and enjoy the rhythm of the music.
14. Write notes if necessary. If the patient can use sign language, inquire into the use of an interpreter.
15. Remember that straining to hear and sorting out background noises are fatiguing.
16. If a patient with dementia also has a hearing aid, be sure it is in during the day. Not hearing can trigger a catastrophic reaction.
17. Provide amplifiers for telephones.

Rationales

Nursing Interventions	Rationales
18. Alert public speakers to the needs of hearing-impaired persons.	
19. Suggest public buildings have individual amplifiers available where lectures, sermons, and group discussions are held.	

▶ **NURSING DIAGNOSIS:** *High Risk for Injury*

Risk Factors
The inability to hear
- smoke/fire alarms
- telephone
- sirens of emergency vehicles

Patient Outcome
The patient will select a method for becoming aware of danger signals.

Nursing Interventions	Rationales
Refer patient to audiologist for advice on alerting and communication devices for hearing-impaired people.	There are alerting and alarm systems that utilize visual, vibro-tactile, or auditory (with increased amplification) stimuli. There are telephone aids and telecommunication devices that decrease the risk for injury and also increase opportunities for socialization.

DISCHARGE PLANNING/CONTINUITY OF CARE
- Assess ability to care for and insert hearing aid.
- Provide name and telephone number of audiologist for hearing aid services.
- Provide information for family regarding communication.

BIBLIOGRAPHY
Haybach, P. J. (1993). Tuning into ototoxicity. *Nursing 93, 23*(6), 34–40.

Ney, D. F. (1993). Cerumen impaction, ear hygiene practices, and hearing acuity. *Geriatric Nursing, 14*(2), 70–73.

O'Rourke, C. M., et al. (1993). *Effectiveness of a hearing screening protocol for the elderly. 14*(2), 66–69.

Ramsdell, D. A. (1970). The psychology of the hard of hearing and the deafened adult. In H. Davis & S. R. Silverman (Eds.) *Hearing and deafness*. New York: Holt, Rinehart, and Winston.

Williams, P. S. (1991). *Hearing loss/information for professionals in the aging network*. National Information Center on Deafness/American-Speech-Language-Hearing Association. Gallaudet University.

$\mathcal{V}$ISION IMPAIRMENT

$\mathbf{V}$ision is normal (emmetropia, 20/20 vision) when rays of light coming from the object at a distance of 20 feet or more are brought to focus on the retina by the lens. Legal blindness is defined as central visual acuity in the better eye of 20/200 or less when using a corrective lens or a visual field of 20° or less at the widest diameter. Persons may be admitted to long-term care facilities because of self-care deficits related to vision impairments. Others may be there because of a co-existing problem. The degree to which an individual can learn self-care skills will depend on cognitive status and whether or not there are other reasons for the self-care deficits.

ETIOLOGIES
- Glaucoma
- Cataract
- Age-related macular degeneration
- Diabetic retinopathy

CLINICAL MANIFESTATIONS
- Glaucoma
    - Narrow angle (acute): pain, blurring of vision, nausea and vomiting
    - Open angle (chronic): clouding, blurring of vision, appearance of halos around lights
- Cataract
    - hazy, fuzzy, or blurred vision
    - dark spots in the field of vision that remain fixed as the eye moves
    - frequent changes in eyeglass prescriptions needed
    - changes in pupil color and problems with light
    - complaints of having a film over the eye
    - frequent blinking in effort to see better
- Age-related macular degeneration
    - blurring
    - distorted vision (loss of central vision)
- Diabetic retinopathy: symptomless until advanced stages

CLINICAL/DIAGNOSTIC FINDINGS
Complete visual examination by ophthalmologist will reveal pathology.

▶ NURSING DIAGNOSIS: *Self-Care Deficit (Feeding)*
Related To vision impairment.

Defining Characteristics
- Observed difficulty with eating skills
- Decreased food intake
- Refusal to eat with others

Patient Outcomes
The patient will
- increase food intake to maintain adequate nutritional status.
- agree to eat in social settings.

Nursing Interventions	Rationales
Sitting at the table, teach the patient to 1. place one hand on the back of the chair and slide it out. 2. make sure the seat is clear by using the free hand to brush back and forth. 3. move to the front of the chair, line the back of the knees against the front of the chair, anchor the chair with one hand, and sit down.	Avoid falls while trying to sit at the table.
To orient self to table setting, teach patient to 1. feel for the edge of the table and adjust position. 2. find his or her plate by reaching forward with both hands and placing fingertips on the top edge of the table. 3. flex the fingers and move hands straight ahead until plate is located. 4. use a trailing technique when reaching for objects—flex the	Prevent spills.

Nursing Interventions	**Rationales**
fingers slightly and keep finger-tips in continuous contact with the table surface as the hand is moved gently forward or laterally on the table.	
Orient patient to location of food on plate: 1. Describe plate like a clock, with meat at 6:00, potatoes at 3:00, vegetables at 9:00. 2. Describe food that is served and position and contents of any side dishes. 3. Place condiments and cream and sugar in the same spot on the table at every meal.	Increase eating enjoyment and confidence in eating.
To eat, teach patient to 1. bend trunk (not head) forward over the plate while eating in case something falls from fork. 2. learn to judge the amount of food on fork by sensing the weight. 3. anchor the plate by pressing down with the knife when cutting with a fork and knife. 4. use a pusher (piece of bread or knife) to pick up food like peas or corn; if the dish has sides, push the food toward the side. 5. shake salt and pepper into hand first rather than directly on the food to prevent overuse. 6. determine the size, shape, and weight of the container before pouring liquids; with one hand, hold the cup with the thumb and middle finger, close to the top with the cup handle close to the tip of the thumb; use index finger as a point of reference to center the pouring container spout; take	Visually impaired persons can remain or regain some independence in the activities of daily living. Individuals who have been vision impaired for several years may have relied on family to do for them, and with the absence of this help, they may be motivated to learn.

Nursing Interventions

Rationales

the pouring container in the other hand and bring the tip of the spout to the side of the cup; with index finger as guide, the spout is centered over the cup; to determine when the cup is full, bend the first joint of the index finger over the edge of the cup. Stop pouring when liquid is felt.

7. handle serving dishes. Teach patient to take the serving dish in right hand, transfer it to left hand, and hold it over the plate.

8. locate the serving utensil by following the rim of the serving dish.

Provide positive reinforcement and assistance as needed.

▶ **NURSING DIAGNOSIS:** *Self-Care Deficit (Bathing, Grooming, Hygiene)*

Related To vision impairment.

Defining Characteristics
• Observed difficulty with bathing, grooming, and hygiene skills
• Disheveled appearance
• Reluctance to ask for assistance

Patient Outcomes
The patient will complete bathing, grooming, and hygiene activities with minimal assistance.

Nursing Interventions

Rationales

Teach the patient to develop a system of organization in the room or house. Have the patient decide where to put belongings and personal care items. Once this is done, make sure the system is maintained.

The patient will be able to locate items without assistance.

Nursing Interventions	Rationales
Set up items needed for bathing and grooming, if necessary, and encourage patient to do as much as possible. Provide assistance when necessary. Give positive feedback.	In the absence of other disabilities, the patient can complete these activities independently if items are available.
Allow patient to choose own clothing. Clothes can be labeled so they can be identified by "feel." Arrange clothes so that coordinated items are together. Tactfully inform if clothing needs attention.	Creativity can increase independence. Even though visually impaired, knowing one is well-groomed boosts self-esteem and gives confidence to socialize with others.

▶ NURSING DIAGNOSIS: *Diversional Activity Deficit*

Related To reluctance to leave room/home due to fear of falling and getting lost.

Defining Characteristics
• Prefers to remain in room
• Refuses to attend activities

Patient Outcomes
The patient will agree to leave room, with assistance, for activities and eating.

Nursing Interventions	Rationales
Monitor the halls and floors frequently for clutter or unnecessary and unexpected items. Never leave doors or drawers partially open.	If patient walks into unexpected barriers, fear is increased.
Teach patient to do the following while walking: 1. Grasp caregiver's arm just above the elbow and have the caregiver remain about two steps ahead. 2. Tell patient if there are steps or curbs or if the incline changes or remains flat and pause before going up or down.	Walking in a strange environment is a fearful situation. To not provide with assistance and instruction is to deprive the patient of enriching experiences and sensory stimulation. The methods used here allow the patient to pick up cues about changes in the walking pattern and facilitate orientation. Describing the

Nursing Interventions

3. Advise patient to put one hand on the rail when walking in hall.
4. Describe landmarks like doors and windows.
5. Suggest using hand to trail the wall and counting doorways.
6. Give directions by telling how many doors to pass before turning right or left.
7. Describe surroundings when in a strange area; use multiple adjectives for colors, textures, and shapes.
8. Orient to room by telling where the bathroom, bed, chairs, dressers, and closet are in relation to the door.
9. Avoid rearranging furniture unless it is necessary, and then reorient patient to the change.
10. Orient to bathroom by describing location of the toilet, sink, toilet paper, and towel racks.

Rationales

environment enables the patient to see in the "mind's eye." Once self-confidence is regained, the patient can assume more independence.

▶ **NURSING DIAGNOSIS:** *Impaired Verbal Communication*

Related To inability to visualize presence of other people.

Defining Characteristics
• Startled reaction when people enter room
• Reluctance to converse with others

Patient Outcome
Patient will be able to visualize presence of other people.

Nursing Interventions

Call by name before entering room, touch lightly, and identify self:
1. Additional information may be needed, such as "I'm your nurse

Rationales

Communication takes many forms. Vision provides many cues for communication, and when these cues are missing, communication is

Nursing Interventions	**Rationales**
on the day shift." Announce departure from room. 2. Be specific when giving directions: "I will put the pill in your right hand" or "I am setting a glass of water on the table to your left." 3. Teach to sign name by placing your index finger at the start of the line. Have the patient locate that finger with the pen and begin writing.	impaired. Anxiety is created when persons silently enter a room without announcing themselves. It is embarrassing for the individual to continue talking and then realize that no one is there listening. Being able to sign checks and documents provides a feeling of being in control.

DISCHARGE PLANNING/CONTINUITY OF CARE
- Provide family with information regarding arrangement of home to facilitate independence.
- Refer to visual rehabilitation consultant.
- Remind to see ophthalmologist as required.

BIBLIOGRAPHY
Agency for Health Care Policy and Research. (1993). *Cataract in adults.* Rockville, MD: U.S. Department of Health and Human Services.

National Institutes of Health. (1989a). *Diabetic retinopathy.* Washington, DC: U.S. Department of Health and Human Services.

National Institutes of Health. (1989b). *Age-related macular degeneration.* Washington, DC: U.S. Department of Health and Human Services.

National Institutes of Health. (1991a). *Cataracts.* Washington, DC: U.S. Department of Health and Human Services.

National Institutes of Health. (1991b). *Glaucoma.* Washington, DC: U.S. Department of Health and Human Services.

Norris, R. M. (1989). Commonsense tips for blind patients. *American Journal of Nursing, 89*(3), 360–361.

Psychosocial Issues

ℰLDER ABUSE

The mistreatment and neglect of the elderly have occurred for hundreds of years. However, it has been only recently that health care professionals have begun to play a role in the detection, management, and prevention of this social phenomenon. There is no universal definition of elder abuse. In general terms, it refers to nonaccidental acts or omissions against an elderly person that cause physical, psychological, or mental harm. This chapter does not address spouse abuse with a long history that has extended into old age and self-abuse related to mental deterioration in a person who lives alone, is unable to care for self, and resists/refuses assistance.

ETIOLOGIES
The etiologies of elder abuse are based on assumptions that have not been corroborated with adequate clinical data. Abuse usually occurs when there is a severely dependent elderly person who is unable to care for physical, financial, or basic personal needs. The caregiver often has problems related to the following:
- alcoholism
- drug addiction
- psychosis
- cognitive impairment
- physical impairment
- perpetuation of violence as a learned behavior
- financial hardship

CLINICAL MANIFESTATIONS
- Physical abuse or neglect (passive or active)
  - bruises, welts, lacerations
  - fractures, burns, rope marks
  - laboratory values indicating overdose or underdose of prescribed medication
  - malnourishment/dehydration
  - pressure ulcers
  - poor personal hygiene

- Sexual abuse
  -unexplained sexually transmitted disease
  -genital infections
- Psychological (mental, verbal) abuse
  -withdrawal, depression
  -agitation
  -signs of infantile behavior
  -expression of ambivalent feelings toward caregivers
- Financial/material abuse
  -suffering from substandard care despite adequate financial resources
  -sudden transfer of assets to others

CLINICAL/DIAGNOSTIC FINDINGS
Confirmed by
- physical assessment/examination
- history/interviews

NOTE: There are many nursing diagnoses that may be associated with elder abuse. This chapter includes psychosocial diagnoses only. Problems related to pressure ulcers, altered nutrition, and other manifestations of neglect are found elsewhere in this text.

▶ NURSING DIAGNOSIS: *Social Isolation*

Related To seclusion imposed by caregiver or self-imposed seclusion due to shame and fear.

Defining Characteristics
- Sad, dull effect
- Uncommunicative
- Withdrawn
- Lack of eye contact

Patient Outcomes
The patient will
- express a sense of self-worth.
- verbalize willingness to be involved with others.

Nursing Interventions	Rationales
Assess 1. physical status 2. cognitive status 3. emotional status 4. social resources 5. financial resources	It is necessary to evaluate the situation thoroughly to determine 1. whether the diagnosis of abuse or neglect is justified. 2. what type of abuse has been committed.

Nursing Interventions	Rationales
	3. which interventions to implement.
Notify appropriate agency if abuse is confirmed (depending on state regulations): 1. Adult Protective Services 2. Department of Aging 3. State Ombudsman (for residents in long-term care facilities)	These agencies can provide health care professionals with the expertise to investigate and further evaluate the circumstances.
Arrange for hospitalization if there are injuries that require treatment or if patient is in danger of immediate injury.	The injury can be treated and the patient will be safe until the investigation is completed and living arrangements can be established.
Assess patient's feelings of helplessness and whether or not patient feels in control of the situation.	Victims of abuse frequently perceive themselves as helpless and unable to prevent or eliminate the abuse that is inflicted. Counseling is needed to alter these perceptions. For the frail elderly, removal from the situation may be the only recourse.
Actively listen to patient's comments and allow patient to ventilate feelings.	Expressing thoughts and feelings is the first step in recognition of the problem and a need for help.
Provide information about support groups that may be beneficial.	The group can offer emotional support and can help eradicate feelings of shame that are often associated with abuse.

▶ NURSING DIAGNOSIS: *Caregiver Role Strain*

Related To
- Complexity of care receiver's needs
- Unpredictability of care receiver's physical/mental condition
- Impaired health of caregiver
- Multiple, sometimes conflicting demands from other sources on caregiver's time and energies

Defining Characteristics
- Lack of financial, emotional, and physical resources

- Lack of knowledge about care receiver's condition and how to provide care
- Family conflicts regarding responsibilities related to caregiving
- Feeling of loss due to physical/mental/emotional changes in care receiver

Patient/Family Outcomes

The patient/family will
- identify the unmet needs of both patient and family.
- identify the responses of the patient/family to the unmet needs.
- arrange for methods to meet the needs of patient/family.

Nursing Interventions	Rationales
Assess caregiver's knowledge concerning health condition of care receiver.	The caregiver may expect the patient to achieve more than what is realistically possible and may have misconceptions about progression of the disease process. The caregiver may be in a state of denial concerning care receiver's condition.
Assess caregiver's physical, mental, and emotional abilities to provide care.	The caregiver may be physically, mentally, or emotionally unable to provide care. Spouses of elderly care receivers are probably also elderly and may have major health problems that prevent them from meeting the responsibilities of caregiving. Children of care receivers may have multiple responsibilities and overextend themselves in their efforts to give care. The need for caregiving often results from a crisis situation that overwhelms the patient and family members. The sudden and unexpected nature of the demands placed upon them has not allowed them to regain their equilibrium. In some cases, friction and conflicts related to caregiving responsibilities stem from a history of dysfunctional relationships.

Nursing Interventions	Rationales
Evaluate need for community resources: homemaker, nursing assistant, professional nursing, therapies, meals, respite, or day care.	Caregiver may be able to manage responsibilities if help is provided on an intermittent basis.
Evaluate environment and caregiving routines to determine if there are alterations that can facilitate caregiving.	Caregivers may be unaware of equipment, procedures, and methods that can ease the workload.
Assess the need for placement in a long-term care facility.	Family members may be reluctant to consider this option because of guilt or lack of knowledge in regard to arranging admission. Frequently caregivers attempt to provide for all of the care receiver's needs after they are physically, mentally, and emotionally exhausted.

▶ NURSING DIAGNOSIS: *Ineffective Family Coping—Disabling*

Related To unexpressed feelings of family members of guilt, resentment, hostility, anger, and despair.

Defining Characteristics
- Disregard for patient's basic needs
- Neglect of patient's required treatments
- Denial of patient's health problems
- Actions detrimental to welfare of patient

Family Outcomes
The family will express understanding of the patient's health problems and care needs.

Nursing Interventions	Rationales
Identify family interactions previous to patient's illness.	There may be long-standing hostilities between family members.
Identify current family interactions.	Accurate assessment of the current situation will provide data for appropriate interventions.

Nursing Interventions	Rationales
Establish rapport with family members.	The family may view health care professionals as interlopers in the situation and refuse to provide information.
Provide honest, brief information during contacts with family members.	Credibility must be established before a trusting relationship develops.
Allow family members to express their feelings without being judgmental.	A myriad of feelings can build up among and between family members during a major crisis. These emotions can be buried because individuals feel they are "bad" for experiencing these feelings. It is an essential part of the healing and coping process to face these feelings.
Work with family to identify coping mechanisms and to evaluate whether or not they are effective.	Individual family members must recognize how they are dealing with the situation and understand whether what they are doing is effective before change can occur.
Serve as liaison between physician and family.	Clarification of the physician's orders regarding treatments, procedures, and medications can increase the family's understanding.
Refer family members to appropriate resources: support groups, counseling, financial services, and health care services.	Family may be unaware of help that is available.

DISCHARGE PLANNING/CONTINUITY OF CARE

If family member is in hospital or long-term care facility:
- Refer to a health care professional who will continue to serve as liaison for the family and who can assess the family situation intermittently.
- If the family member is in the hospital and will have ongoing health care needs for a lengthy period, temporary admission to a long-term care facility may need to be suggested.

If the family member is home:
- Continue with home care services until the crisis is resolved or until family members are able to provide for patient's needs.

BIBLIOGRAPHY

Aravanis, S. C., et al. (1992). *Diagnostic and treatment guidelines on elder abuse and neglect.* Chicago: American Medical Association.

Douglass, R. L. (1992). *Domestic mistreatment of the elderly.* Washington, DC: American Association of Retired People.

Mowbray, C. A. (1989). Shedding light on elder abuse. *Journal of Gerontological Nursing, 15*(10), 20–24.

$\mathcal{D}$EPRESSION

Depression describes a syndrome that includes a cluster of physiological, psychosocial, and cognitive manifestations. The onset is insidious, and in the elderly, the symptoms may go unrecognized in the presence of multiple, co-occurring physical problems. Depressed persons feel alone and isolated and suffer a greatly diminished quality of life. There are two types of clinical depression. Major depression can occur for the first time at any age. It may occur only once in a lifetime or it may recur several times. Bipolar disorder (manic-depressive illness) is believed to be inherited, is characterized by severe mood swings, usually starts in young adulthood, and may persist throughout life. Both types of depression affect all aspects of the individual's life and both require professional treatment.

ETIOLOGIES
There are no known specific causes of depression. There are several risk factors associated with depression:
- being female
- being unmarried, particularly widowed
- experiencing stressful life events
- lacking supportive social network
- co-occurrence of physical medical conditions
- medication
- alcohol
- living in a long-term care facility or other residential setting

CLINICAL MANIFESTATIONS
- Changes in
  - appetite
  - weight
  - sleep habits
- Digestive problems
- Sexual problems
- Headaches
- Motor agitation or retardation

- Fatigue and loss of energy
- Depressed or irritable mood
- Loss of interest or pleasure in usual activities
- Feelings of worthlessness, excessive guilt
- Difficulty with thinking or concentrating
- Suicidal thinking

CLINICAL/DIAGNOSTIC FINDINGS
- Physical examination: to determine if a general medical disorder is the cause of the depressive symptoms
- Health history
- Family history
- Mental health evaluation

▶ NURSING DIAGNOSIS: *Fatigue*

Related To inability to deal with overwhelming emotional demands.

Defining Characteristics
- Verbalization of inundating and continuing lack of energy
- Inability to maintain usual activities

Patient Outcomes
The patient will
- verbalize feelings of increased energy.
- gradually resume usual routines and activities.

Nursing Interventions	Rationales
Assess for signs of physical basis for fatigue: infection, pain, altered nutritional status, and shortness of breath upon exertion.	In the elderly patient, physiological distress may precipitate fatigue.
Administer treatment for underlying physiological problem.	Correction of underlying problem will decrease fatigue.
Provide opportunity to ventilate feelings about past and present life experiences.	Ventilation of feelings reduces the amount of emotional energy that is required by internalizing emotions.
Plan and encourage intake of nourishing and an appetizing diet.	Elderly persons may acquire unhealthy eating habits and suffer fatigue related to undernutrition.

Nursing Interventions	Rationales
Assist with scheduling activities of choice interspersed with periods of rest. Establish small goals for completing activities. Introduce new activities as goals are accomplished.	A structured schedule with goals to meet provides direction and a reason for adhering to the schedule. Variety may increase motivation and outlook.
Include physical exercise in the schedule.	Physical activity increases energy levels and reduces fatigue.
Establish a therapeutic, psychological environment.	The appropriate use of art, music, color, and furnishings and the right degree of sensory stimulation can lift the spirits and increase psychological comfort.

▶ NURSING DIAGNOSIS: *Hopelessness*

Related To
- Failing or deteriorating physiological or psychosocial condition
- Long-term stress
- Enforcing of learned helplessness

Defining Characteristics
- Lack of affect
- Passivity
- Decreased verbalization, frequent sighing
- Lack of involvement in all aspects of life

Patient Outcomes
The patient will
- verbalize feelings and ideas.
- participate in activities of daily living.
- demonstrate control over self and the environment.

Nursing Interventions	Rationales
Assess for verbal or nonverbal signs of suicidal thoughts/intent.	Prevention of suicide attempt is dependent on identification of risk factors.
Assess for underlying physiological conditions that can cause feelings of	Interventions can be established to increase physical comfort and to

Nursing Interventions	Rationales
hopelessness: progressive disease processes, terminal illness, unrelenting pain, or the inability to manage activities of daily living.	assist in adaptation to an altered life-style.
Establish a therapeutic relationship.	A sense of trust facilitates expression of feelings and increases willingness to comply with interventions.
Evaluate relationships and assist to identify persons who can serve as a support system. Include these persons in care-planning process (with approval of patient).	The presence of significant other(s) decreases feelings of isolation and activates interest outside of self. Involvement in care planning encourages significant others to participate in appropriate interventions.
Involve in activities of daily living, providing assistance and modifying environment as necessary. Give opportunities for making simple nonfail decisions. Give positive feedback for accomplishments.	Performing within the realm of current ability and making successful decisions increases self-confidence. Positive feedback reinforces the behavior. Underlying physiological causes for self-care deficits require assistance of caregiver and modification of environment to avoid further increasing feelings of hopelessness and defeat.
Plan activities and establish small goals to ensure success. Present greater challenges as goals are met. Give positive feedback.	As success is experienced, the willingness to take risks by accepting new challenges increases self-confidence and enables the patient to reach beyond minimum levels of achievement.

▶ **NURSING DIAGNOSIS:** *Diversional Activity Deficit*

Related To fatigue and feelings of hopelessness.

Defining Characteristics
- Loss of interest in previous activities
- Refusal to participate in usual activities
- Prefers to be alone

Patient Outcomes

The patient will
- verbalize interest in previous activities.
- participate in activities of choice.

Nursing Interventions	Rationales
Assess past hobbies, interests, and pastimes.	Data can guide selection of activities from which patient can choose.
Assess physiological and cognitive status.	Co-occurring medical problems may limit participation in previous interests, and substitutions will need to be selected.
Conduct one-on-one staff interactions to invite, plan, and schedule attendance at activities of choice. Schedule volunteer to visit and guide solitary activities: read aloud, write letters, walk with patient outside, and converse about current events.	Individualized attention and interaction increases feelings of self worth. One-on-one activities can generate interest outside of the self and increase feelings of normalcy.
Guide in selection of activities that are failproof and noncompetitive.	Experiencing success provides incentive to continue with activities. The need to compete increases the risk of failure and requires unavailable emotional energies.
Guide in selection of nonthreatening group activities such as musical presentations.	Social interaction is provided in a situation where patient does not experience stress due to the need to perform or compete.
Encourage reminiscence.	Reflecting and talking about life experiences validates self-worth and confirms the purpose of one's being.

▶ NURSING DIAGNOSIS: *High Risk for Self-Directed Violence*

Risk Factors
- Verbalization of feelings of unrelenting hopelessness
- Increased anxiety levels
- Increased motor activity

- Unresolved grief
- Verbalization of suicidal thoughts
- Caucasian race
- Male gender
- Living alone
- Advanced age
- History of prior suicide attempts, family history of suicide attempts, and family history of substance abuse

Patient Outcomes

The patient will
- avoid suicidal behaviors.
- increase satisfying interactions with others.
- verbalize increased feelings of self-worth.

Nursing Interventions	Rationales
Monitor for sudden changes in behavior and for signs of increased anxiety (pacing, wringing of hands, increased smoking).	Nonverbal clues may be the only indication of suicidal behaviors.
Monitor for abrupt and unexpected changes in mood that reflect feelings of suddenly being at peace with oneself.	A decision to terminate one's life as a way to find peace may result in a calmness and composure previously not observed.
Investigate whether patient is taking medication as ordered.	When appropriate medication is prescribed and taken as ordered, suicidal thoughts go away. Discontinuing of medication may generate suicidal thoughts.
Actively listen while encouraging verbalizations of negative feelings.	Anxiety may be alleviated. Knowing that someone cares may reduce suicidal thoughts.
Assess spiritual and religious beliefs.	Religious practices and pastoral counseling may assuage feelings of hopelessness.
Assess previous coping skills.	Identification of previous coping patterns and responses provides knowledge for dealing with current situation.
Arrange a safe environment.	Removal of potentially dangerous objects reduces the risk of self-destruction.

DISCHARGE PLANNING/CONTINUITY OF CARE

- Reinforce the need for taking medication as prescribed. Instruct patient to report any side effects of the medication.
- Reinforce the need to keep appointments with primary care provider.
- Advise the patient to keep a daily activity record that documents the taking of medications, symptoms experienced, and activities completed.
- Provide a local crisis line number for the patient to use if depression is overwhelming and other sources of help are not available.

BIBLIOGRAPHY

Browning, M. A. (1990). Depression. In M. O. Hogstel (Ed.), *Geropsychiatric Nursing,* (pp. 130–176). St. Louis, MO: The C. V. Mosby Co.

Keane, S. M., & Sells, S. (1990). Recognizing depression in the elderly. *Journal of Gerontological Nursing, 16*(1), 21–25.

National Institutes of Health. (1991). *Diagnosis and treatment of depression in late life. Consensus statement.* Bethesda, MD: U.S. Department of Health and Human Services.

Newbern, V. B. (1992). Failure to thrive: A growing concern in the elderly. *Journal of Gerontological Nursing, 18*(8), 21–25.

U.S. Department of Health and Human Services. (April 1993). *Depression is a treatable illness.* Rockville, MD: Public Health Service, Agency for Health Care Policy and Research.

SEXUALITY AND THE OLDER ADULT WITH CHRONIC ILLNESS

Sexuality is a life-long need. In spite of the myths surrounding the sexual behavior of the elderly, they can be and are sexually active. While there are numerous aging changes that affect sexual functioning, both males and females are capable of orgasmic sexual performance. Sexuality encompasses the realm of all that is unique in the maleness and femaleness of each person. It is the ability to give and receive love and to share intimacy. Many older adults find pleasure and satisfaction in emotional and physical closeness. The relationship may or may not include coitus. Despite the interest and desire to maintain an active sex life, there may be medical or psychosocial problems that present barriers to pursuing such activity. This chapter is directed toward those problems. Sensitivity is a necessary prerequisite for sexual counseling of the elderly. Most individuals in this age group have had enough sexual experience to know what is acceptable and pleasing. Some aged persons may have retired from sexual activity and are happy with that decision.

ETIOLOGIES
- Medical conditions
- Medications
- Lack of a significant other
- Lack of privacy

CLINICAL MANIFESTATIONS
- Expressions of feelings of loneliness
- Impaired physical mobility
- Absence of significant other

CLINICAL/DIAGNOSTIC FINDINGS
Sexual history indicates
- disability that interferes with sexual relationships.

- misperceptions of own sexuality prior to medical problem and at current time.
- medications that interfere with sexual response.
- unwilling or unavailable partner.
- lack of knowledge concerning sexuality.

▶ **NURSING DIAGNOSIS:** *Altered Sexuality Patterns*

Related To change in body image due to health problem.

Defining Characteristics
Expressed dissatisfaction with body image and inability to resume relationship due to fear of rejection by partner. This may be the result of
- surgical removal of a body part, such as an extremity, breast, or testicles.
- surgery resulting in altered body function, such as colostomy or catheter insertion.
- trauma resulting in scarring and deformity from burns, fractures, and lacerations.
- treatments that alter appearance, such as loss of hair.

Even though appearance is unchanged, body image can be affected by changes in functional ability: mobility and ability to resume former roles.

Patient Outcomes
The patient will
- verbalize self-acceptance.
- verbalize willingness to seek information concerning condition.
- verbalize readiness to pursue relationship with partner.

Nursing Interventions	Rationales
Assess signs of grieving. Encourage patient to verbalize feelings and concerns about current situation.	The patient may still be working through the grieving process. Indications of prolonged grieving or depression require intervention.
Assess mobility, endurance, and strength.	Patient may have deficits in these areas as a result of the medical condition. These deficits will need to be addressed as they may affect body image and interfere with sexual activity.
Complete a sexual history.	Data may indicate that 1. a sexual problem existed prior to the current illness.

Nursing Interventions	Rationales
	2. the patient and/or the partner subconsciously wishes to withdraw from sexual activity.
Assess appearance, grooming, and hygiene. Assess knowledge concerning opportunities for cosmetic adaptations to body changes.	Good hygiene and grooming and attractive physical appearance increase sex appeal. Prostheses for missing body parts, wigs to replace hair loss, and cosmetics to cover scarring can increase self-confidence.
Assess interactions of patient and partner.	Partner may be 1. reinforcing patient's negative perceptions of self. 2. unsure of what patient is expecting in terms of support and assistance. 3. fearful that any physical contact will cause injury to patient. 4. lacking knowledge of patient's condition and prognosis.
Establish rapport with patient/partner and encourage them to verbalize feelings and concerns. Avoid being judgmental and assure that negative feelings are not bad. Provide privacy and encourage open communication between patient and partner. Encourage partner to treat patient as a normal person and not as an invalid.	Exploration of feelings and concerns can provide a foundation for physical and emotional intimacy.
Develop interventions based on assessment data: 1. counseling for patient and/or significant other 2. suggestions for adapting sexual activity to current situation (see interventions later in chapter for specific medical problems) 3. arranging for prosthetic and cosmetic consultants	The presence of physical or psychosocial barriers to sexual activity may require nursing intervention to facilitate the relationship of the involved parties.

▶ NURSING DIAGNOSIS: *Sexual Dysfunction*

Related To fear of having sexual relations due to recent myocardial infarction.

Defining Characteristics
- Verbalization of problem
- Perceived limitation imposed by disease

Patient Outcomes
The patient will
- verbalize understanding of body function.
- verbalize diminished fear related to sexual activity.
- resume satisfying sexual relationship.

Nursing Interventions	Rationales
Assess current cardiovascular condition. Determine information that physician related to patient/partner.	Assure that sexual activity will not trigger dangerous manifestations.
Assess knowledge of patient and partner concerning patient's health history and current status.	Inaccurate perceptions may need to be resolved before teaching can be initiated.
Assess medication regime.	Some antihypertensive medications and tricyclic antidepressants can affect libido.
Assure patient that 1. sexual activity can be safely resumed with familiar partner in 8–14 weeks. 2. blood pressure, pulse, and respirations will increase, but not enough to be harmful. 3. position during intercourse has little effect on physical energy requirements.	After myocardial infarction, both the patient and partner may be fearful that sexual activity will result in further heart damage.
Advise patient 1. to avoid sexual activity after a heavy meal. 2. to avoid excessive alcohol intake. 3. that psychic stress may result from sexual activity with a new	Evidence suggests that myocardial infarction during sexual activity can occur after heavy consumption of food and/or alcohol. Research indicates that sexual activity after myocardial infarction is safe when

Nursing Interventions	Rationales
partner, in unfamiliar circumstances, or with new techniques.	performed with a familiar partner using familiar techniques in familiar surroundings. Changes from what the patient is accustomed to may trigger psychic stress that can affect physical function.
Advise male patients and their partners that temporary impotence may occur as a result of anxiety about resuming sexual activity. Advise to seek medical assistance or counseling if several episodes occur.	Temporary impotence is not uncommon, but it may become permanent if it continues to recur and intervention is not sought. An awareness that this is not unusual may prevent further anxiety should it occur.
Advise female patients and their partners that the 8–14 weeks without sexual activity can result in vaginal changes including narrowing and shrinking of the walls. The first attempts at sexual intercourse may be uncomfortable and somewhat painful. Resumption of sexual activity will resolve the problem.	Knowledge of these changes can alert the partner to be considerate and thoughtful during sexual activity.

▶ **NURSING DIAGNOSIS:** *Sexual Dysfunction*

Related To dyspnea during sexual activity due to chronic obstructive pulmonary disease.

Defining Characteristics
• Verbalization of problem
• Observance of dyspnea and wheezing during physical exertion

Patient Outcomes
The patient will
• express knowledge of interventions to facilitate sexual activity.
• express acceptance of alternative sexual practices.

Nursing Interventions	Rationales
Advise patient to plan for sexual activity when energy levels are highest, generally in late morning or midafternoon. Advise pacing activity and going slow.	Planning for sexual activity when there is adequate time allows for relaxation and reduced stress. Mornings may need to be avoided as secretions accumulate during sleep.
Suggest the following: 1. pursed-lip or diaphragmatic breathing 2. if the patient has oxygen that it be used at the prescribed rate during sexual activity 3. waiting 30–60 min after inhaler use or nebulizer treatment before sexual activity	These interventions increase activity tolerance.
Suggest a regular exercise program such as walking every day.	Increasing activity tolerance will improve sexual activity.
Advise using positions that reduce pressure on chest such as side-lying or sitting.	Pressure and weight on the chest increase breathing difficulty.
Advise patient that prolonged kissing or oral sex may need to be avoided.	These activities may increase dyspnea, causing panic.
Maintain room temperature of 68–72 F with 40% humidity.	Environmental temperature affects oxygen consumption.
Advise male patient to use a bronchodilator before sexual activity to avoid coughing.	Coughing can cause loss of erection, but it can be regained.
Suggest that intimacy and sexual play can be as rewarding as coitus.	The pressure to achieve orgasm may increase performance anxiety, resulting in dyspnea and further anxiety.

▶ **NURSING DIAGNOSIS:** *Sexual Dysfunction*

Related To pain due to arthritic joint changes.

Defining Characteristics
• Verbalization of problem

Patient Outcomes

The patient will verbalize understanding of interventions to enhance sexual activity.

Nursing Interventions	Rationales
Evaluate patient's perceptions of body image.	Persons with joint deformities (especially those related to rheumatoid arthritis) may have an altered body image due to visible changes in joints.
Evaluate medication regime.	Steroids may affect libido.
Advise patient that arthritis does not usually affect physiological sexual function, including the capacity for arousal and fulfillment. Adaptations and a considerate partner can enhance a sexual relationship.	Allay possible concerns of the patient regarding sexual capacity and abilities.
Advise patient to plan ahead for sexual activity: 1. Take a warm bath or shower. 2. Do active or active assistive range-of-motion exercises 30 min before activity in all joints. Avoid exercising to the point of pain or fatigue. 3. Massage joints gently. 4. Take analgesic or nonsteroidal anti-inflammatory drugs (NSAID) 30 min before activity.	Ease joint stiffness and pain, facilitating sexual activity.
Suggest experimenting with various positions for sexual activity. Place pillows under affected joints.	Utilize positions that place minimal stress upon stiff and painful joints.
Suggest the use of satin sheets.	Satin sheets can facilitate movement.

▶ NURSING DIAGNOSIS: *Sexual Dysfunction*

Related To altered thought processes due to dementia.

Defining Characteristics
- Verbalization of problem by significant other
- Disorientation and short-term memory deficit of patient

Patient Outcomes
The significant other will verbalize satisfaction with relationship.

Nursing Interventions	Rationales
Assess patient's cognitive status.	Alzheimer's disease and other dementias in the early stages do not generally affect sexual function. As the disease progresses, impaired judgment may be reflected in hypersexuality or interest in sexual activity at inappropriate times.
Discuss with partner feelings and concerns about patient and their relationship.	The partner may have ambivalent feelings related to a blurred distinction between caregiver/lover roles. Personality changes in the patient may be reflected in anger and paranoia directed toward the partner, diminishing the partner's romantic feelings toward the patient.
Encourage patient and partner to 1. set aside times for privacy, quiet, and relaxation. 2. express affection and intimacy openly and honestly. 3. avoid setting full orgasmic experience as the goal for these occasions. 4. enjoy coitus when both partners are emotionally and physically receptive.	Persons with dementia are affected by the environment and by the feelings of the people around them even if these feelings are unexpressed. A quiet environment and a relaxed partner can facilitate sexual activity.
Encourage the partner to arrange for occasional respite care of the patient.	Partners of persons with a dementia are at high risk for caregiver role strain. The continuing stress of providing for the patient will eventually erode all aspects of the relationship.

► NURSING DIAGNOSIS: *Sexual Dysfunction*

Related To changes in sex role and dependency in self-care due to hemiplegia resulting from stroke.

Defining Characteristics
- Male: verbalization of inability to achieve erection
- Both sexes: verbalization of decline in sexual responsiveness

Patient Outcomes
The patient may express satisfaction with sexuality.

Nursing Interventions	Rationales
Arrange for evaluation to determine whether impotence is physiological or psychogenic.	Intervention is selected depending on the cause of impotence.
Complete a functional assessment for activities of daily living. Arrange for rehabilitative/restorative interventions to increase functional abilities.	Dependency on the partner for activities of daily living correlates with decreased sexual activity. Having the partner assist with toileting activities can be distressing to the patient, altering sex role identity.
Assess communication abilities. Arrange for speech therapy if necessary.	Communication is essential to a satisfying sexual relationship. Persons with impaired communication related to aphasia or verbal apraxia may benefit from speech therapy or be taught alternative methods of communication.
Discuss with patient and partner role changes that have occurred as a result of the patient's stroke. Suggest the use of community services to relieve the spouse of some responsibilities.	Changes in marital roles may result in dissatisfied sexual inactivity, particularly if the healthy partner is carrying additional responsibilities.
Discuss the feelings of both individuals regarding life-style and role changes resulting from stroke. Arrange for counseling if necessary.	Changes in mental status, fear of having another stroke, and financial concerns result in loss of self-esteem and can cause fixation on a sick role. The spouse may adopt a custodial role, infantilizing the patient.

Nursing Interventions	Rationales
Suggest positions for sexual activity that are adapted to the physical abilities of the patient.	Facilitate sexual activity.

▶ **NURSING DIAGNOSIS:** *Altered Sexuality Patterns*

Related To lack of privacy due to residence in nursing care facility.

Defining Characteristics
• Verbalization of problem

Patient Outcomes
The patient will verbalize satisfying relationship with partner.

Nursing Interventions

Nursing Interventions	
Perform a sexual assessment on all residents admitted to the facility.	Completing an assessment recognizes sexuality as an ongoing need that can be addressed openly and honestly. The interest of the resident in sexual activity is recognized, and high-risk factors for sexual dysfunction are identified.
Assess patient's living arrangements at the facility.	The Residents' Rights as developed by federal legislation require that married couples may share the same room if both partners are in agreement and if there are no medical reasons for separation.
Meet with both residents individually and then together to discuss their wishes concerning the relationship.	There are situations when one spouse does not wish to resume or continue the sexual relationship. The conflict of desires may need to be addressed if the other spouse is not in agreement. New relationships may be established among residents not married to each other. Identify fears of either person concerning outcome of the relationship. Assure that

Nursing Interventions	Rationales
	neither person has been coerced by the other to participate in the relationship.
Develop a plan of care that provides for the sexual needs of the resident and partner: 1. Consider safety and the prevention of infectious disease. 2. Consider the rights of other residents. 3. Provide counseling for adaptations required for problems related to medical condition. 4. Arrange for uninterrupted privacy.	Initiating and/or maintaining a loving relationship in a nursing facility requires a cooperative effort on the part of the staff.
Arrange for staff education regarding sexuality and the elderly.	Staff members frequently have false perceptions and beliefs about sexuality and aging. Staff needs to be comfortable and knowledgeable about the topic if the needs of the residents are to be met.
Arrange for time away from the facility if the medical condition of both partners permits.	Lack of opportunities for intimacy presents a hardship for spouses in the community when their partners are residing in a long-term care facility. Being at home together for even a few hours is satisfying and rewarding to both individuals. When both partners reside in a facility, it may be beneficial to spend a night or a few hours in a local hotel.

DISCHARGE PLANNING/CONTINUITY OF CARE
- Refer to sex therapist or mental health counselor for more intensive counseling if necessary.

BIBLIOGRAPHY

Burgener, S., & Logan, G. (1989). Sexuality concerns of the poststroke patient. *Rehabilitation Nursing, 14*(4), 178–181, 195.

Hahn, K. (1989). Sexuality and copd. *Rehabilitation Nursing, 14*(4), 191–195.

Seidl, A., et al. (1991). Understanding the effects of a myocardial infarction on sexual functioning: A basis for sexual counseling. *Rehabilitation Nursing, 16*(5), 255–264.

Smedley, G. (1991). Addressing sexuality in the elderly. *Rehabilitation Nursing, 16*(1), 9–11.

Wallace, M. (1992). Management of sexual relationships among elderly residents of long-term care facilities. *Geriatric Nursing, 13*(6), 308–311.

$\mathcal{T}$ERMINAL ILLNESS

The death of a patient is a common occurrence in the practice of geronto-logical nursing. The elderly die in the same manner as younger patients; suddenly and unexpectedly or after a long bout with a terminal illness. Some experience a progressive deterioration that terminates in death. Death is often a welcome release to the elderly who have lost everything that was dear to them. A terminal illness is defined as one that is incurable, irre-versible, and expected to end in death. The diagnosis may be made months or years before death occurs. The hospice definition usually states that death is expected within 6 months.

ETIOLOGIES
- Cancer
- Autoimmune disease
- Cardiovascular disease
- Pulmonary disease
- Alzheimer's or other dementia
- Acquired immunodeficiency syndrome (AIDS)

CLINICAL MANIFESTATIONS
Progressive decline in
- self-care skills
- cognition
- mobility
- nutritional status

CLINICAL/DIAGNOSTIC FINDINGS
Dependent on medical diagnosis

▶ NURSING DIAGNOSIS: *Pain*
Related To disease progression:
- growth of malignant tumor
- metastasis of tumor
- diminished tissue perfusion
- inflammatory process

Defining Characteristics

- Verbalization of pain
- Facial expressions and body posture
- Physical and social withdrawal
- Changes in sleep patterns
- Anorexia
- Inability to continue previous activities

Patient Outcomes

The patient will verbalize relief from pain.

Nursing Interventions	Rationales
Administer pain medication q4h around the clock.	Maintaining a consistent blood level of pain-relieving medication will prevent the onset of pain. Pain may get out of control if medication is given only after the pain is severe and it is then more difficult to alleviate.
Assess the patient to determine the effectiveness of the medication. If the patient suffers episodes of pain, ask the patient to rate the pain on a scale of 1 to 10 with 1 as being mild pain and 10 as the worst pain ever experienced.	Pain is a subjective, personal experience. The patient is the best judge of the severity of the pain. At the onset of terminal illness, the patient may be receiving a nonsteroidal anti-inflammatory drug (NSAID) or acetaminophen with codeine. As the disease state progresses, morphine may be needed to alleviate the pain.
Indicate acceptance of the patient's complaints of pain.	Acceptance and belief of the patient's complaints builds trust and rapport with the patient. If short-acting opiates are given at ineffective dosing intervals because of disbelief of patient's complaints, pseudo-addiction can occur. Because of inadequate pain treatment, the patient may exhibit signs of psychological dependency and resort to bizarre behavior to prove that medication is needed.

Nursing Interventions	Rationales
Monitor for signs of sudden, acute, temporary pain.	Treatments or procedures may trigger the occurrence of breakthrough pain. Adjusted doses of the medication or supplemental medication should be administered as soon as possible. If the precipitating factor is known, administer the medication 30–60 min before the event.
Use nonpharmacologic techniques with the medication. Consult with the patient regarding the use of progressive relaxation techniques or guided imagery. Transcutaneous electrical nerve stimulation (TENS) may be effective in some situations.	These techniques do not replace pain medication but can augment their effectiveness. Relaxation can improve the patient's emotional status.
Monitor bowel elimination.	Constipation is a common side effect of analgesia. Prevention of constipation eliminates another source of physical discomfort.

▶ NURSING DIAGNOSIS: *Altered Nutrition—Less Than Body Requirements*

Related To loss of appetite due to medication, treatments, disease process, or impaired swallowing.

Defining Characteristics
- Loss of weight
- Observed disinterest or inability to eat

Patient Outcomes
The patient will
- participate in meal planning and food selection.
- maintain a desirable weight.
- be able to ingest food without aspiration.

Nursing Interventions	Rationales
Give the patient suggestions for foods that may be more appetizing and easier to swallow: 1. drinking milk and eating milk products 2. avoiding foods with temperature extremes, foods that are spicy or acidic and foods that are hard, crunchy, or coarse 3. using liquids such as gravies, sauces, or mayonnaise that can be added to solid foods	These suggestions may be helpful because 1. milk and milk products coat the mucous membrane, making eating more comfortable. 2. these types of foods may be difficult to chew and to swallow. 3. addition of liquids facilitates swallowing.
Talk with the family to see if there are special foods they can bring in that the patient likes.	The family may bring in foods that are not normally part of the hospital/nursing facility menu. Aside from the nutritional value, food has many attributes. The memories or meaning associated with a certain food may have significant value for the patient.
Consult with the dietician or the caregiver in the home: 1. Prepare double-strength milk by mixing dry skim milk with liquid milk instead of water and mix instant breakfast drinks with the double-strength milk. 2. Use evaporated, condensed, or double-strength milk to make casseroles, puddings, milk shakes, and soups. 3. Add cheese, cream cheese, and whipped cream to appropriate foods. 4. Add margarine to sandwiches and cooked vegetables. Add eggs, meat, poultry, and fish to salads, casseroles, and sandwiches. Give commercially prepared protein-rich supplements between meals.	Calories and nutrients are increased without adding quantity to the meals.

Nursing Interventions	Rationales
Include high-fiber foods that are easy to swallow, such as cooked prunes, prune juice, and whole-grain cereals with milk.	Constipation can become a problem as a result of medication and inactivity.
Prepare the patient for mealtime and provide an appetite-stimulating environment. Arrange for pain medication to be administered 30–60 min before meals.	Eating is more enjoyable if the patient is physically comfortable and is in an environment that is quiet and calm.
Assess oral mucosa daily and assist patient with careful and thorough mouth care at least twice daily. Use a soft-bristle toothbrush and non-irritating toothpaste and instruct patient to rinse with a solution of 500 mL water, $\frac{1}{2}$ teaspoon salt, and $\frac{1}{2}$ teaspoon sodium bicarbonate q4h. Avoid the use of glycerine and lemon juice swabs, which may irritate the oral tissues. Avoid commercial mouth washes containing alcohol. Lubricate patient's lips with cocoa butter or lip balm.	Protein malnutrition can cause stomatitis, resulting in painful ulcerations.
Discuss with the patient/family their feelings regarding the use of a feeding tube if the patient reaches the point of being unable to eat. (This may be indicated on the Advance Directives.)	While this may not become an issue, the patient/family need to be aware that it is a possibility. If the patient's choice is not indicated on Advance Directives, the family/patient may need to make that decision in the future.

▶ NURSING DIAGNOSIS: *Impaired Physical Mobility*

Related To:
- Loss of endurance
- Weakness
- Problems caused by disease process

Defining Characteristics
- Inability to purposefully move within the physical environment

Patient Outcomes

The patient will be free of the complications associated with immobility.

Nursing Interventions	Rationales
Plan a schedule for repositioning the patient at least q2h. Do skin inspection and give a back-and-joint massage with each change.	Changing position alleviates joint stiffness, enhances circulation, and provides a different visual focus. Observe for Stage I pressure ulcers during the skin inspection to implement immediate treatment if necessary. The massage increases physical comfort and induces relaxation.
Do passive or active assistive range-of-motion (PROM, AAROM) twice a day.	Range-of-motion exercises prevent joint stiffness and contracture formation. Contractures increase the risk of impaired skin integrity.
Get the patient out of bed once or twice each day if possible. Transfer the patient with a transfer belt (if patient can bear weight on one or both legs) or mechanical lifter if necessary. Position the patient in a recliner or other chair that is comfortable.	Getting the patient out of bed allows for additional position changes, facilitates socialization, and increases sensory stimulation. Using a transfer belt or mechanical lifter decreases the risk of injury to patient and staff.

▶ NURSING DIAGNOSIS: *High Risk for Impaired Skin Integrity*

Risk Factors

- Physical immobility
- Moisture from skin excretions
- Possible incontinence
- Nutritional status

Patient Outcomes

The patient will remain free of impaired skin integrity.

Nursing Interventions	Rationales
(See Pressure Ulcer, page 13.)	

▶ NURSING DIAGNOSIS: *Social Isolation*

Related To:
- Altered physical appearance
- Altered mental status
- Terminal status

Defining Characteristics
- Absence of supportive significant others
- Sad, dull affect

Patient Outcomes
The patient will
- express increased sense of self-worth.
- be involved in activities of level of ability and desire.
- express acceptance of what cannot be changed.

Nursing Interventions	Rationales
Assess patient for 1. feelings about self and significant others. 2. feelings of control over situation. 3. feeling of hope/hopelessness. 4. use of effective coping skills.	Assessing the patient's feelings helps determine the validity of the nursing diagnosis. The nurse's perception of the patient's isolation may not be accurate if the patient chooses to be alone and is more content with fewer people around. If the isolation is not self-imposed, the patient can be guided to using coping skills that have proven effective in the past.
Strive to establish a therapeutic nurse-patient relationship.	It is not uncommon for friends and perhaps family members to distance themselves from a loved one who is dying. A therapeutic relationship with the nurse will build a sense of trust within the patient. In some situations, the nurse may be the only person the patient will be able to talk to about dying.
Identify support systems and significant others in the patient's life.	Persons who are important to the patient may wish to be supportive but lack direction and confidence in what their actions should be at this point. The patient may be

Nursing Interventions	Rationales
	reluctant to ask for their support. By identifying and assessing the situation, the nurse can determine whether or not it would be appropriate to serve as a facilitator.
Involve the patient with a suitable support group if possible.	The patient may be able to receive emotional support from others who are experiencing the same circumstances.

▶ NURSING DIAGNOSIS: *Altered Family Processes*

Related To changes in family structure and responsibilities and to uncertainty of the future.

Defining Characteristics
- Family's/patient's inability to express and accept feelings of each other
- Failure to send and receive clear messages
- Inability to request or accept help
- Inability to make decisions

Patient/Family Outcomes
The patient/family will
- develop effective, open communication.
- make satisfying decisions.
- seek and accept help when necessary.

Nursing Interventions	Rationales
Identify the structure of the family.	In many families, each member has a role. The relationship of each child to a parent is different and unique. The spouse who is viewed as being the more dependent person in the relationship may prove to be the strongest and most capable when necessary. Becoming familiar with the family structure provides opportunity to develop effective interventions.

Nursing Interventions	Rationales
Actively listen to the family's and patient's expressions of feelings in a nonjudgmental manner.	Families of terminally ill patients experience many emotions including anger, guilt, resentment, anxiety, and fear. They may be shameful of such feelings and be hesitant to express them. It is important that they be reassured that these feelings are normal and acceptable.
Identify resources or support systems outside the family that may provide assistance for emotional support, physical assistance for caring for the patient at home, financial consultation, and spiritual guidance.	Terminal illness of a family member presents many issues that may require the assistance of other professionals.
Invite the family (and patient if possible) to the care plan conference.	The family will be able to identify members of the interdisciplinary team and will develop a trusting relationship with the staff. This can facilitate communication between the care team, the patient, and the family.
Ask the patient/family about their decisions regarding Advance Directives. (Patient's should be asked this question upon admission to the health care system: hospital, nursing home, hospice, or home care.) If Advance Directives have not been established by the patient, discuss with the patient/family the kind of decisions that may need to be made regarding the patient's health care.	It is beneficial for the patient and family to look ahead and establish plans that will affect health care and decisions and financial arrangements. The patient can gain a sense of control in knowing that these wishes will be carried out by family and health care professionals. (See Table 31.1, page 332.)

▶ NURSING DIAGNOSIS: *Hopelessness*

Related To:
- Deteriorating condition
- Spiritual distress
- Isolation

Defining Characteristics
- Decreased verbalization
- Decreased affect
- Increased passivity

Patient Outcomes
The patient will find meaning and direction in life.

Nursing Interventions	Rationales
Talk with the patient to determine if there are underlying fears or anxieties that are causing the feeling of hopelessness.	The patient may be fearful of suffering intolerable pain before death.
Develop a trusting relationship with the patient. Discuss the plans for pain management. Tell the patient what the staff will do and teach the patient what to do to prevent/alleviate pain.	Honest communication and trust allows the patient to focus on other aspects of living if fears of pain are allayed.
Find out if Advance Directives have been written. Assure that the patient's wishes will be carried out and that the patient will be allowed to die with dignity. If directives have not been written, suggest to the patient/family the need for such action.	Patients often fear dying more than death. Fear may be related to the manner in which one will die. In the terminal stages of illness, it is not realistic or kind to hope for a cure. Hope should be based on physical, emotional, and mental comfort during the final days.
Listen to the patient, accepting what is said without being judgmental. Look for nonverbal cues. Encourage reminiscing and communication with loved ones. Arrange for uninterrupted, private visits with the spouse.	The patient may have "unfinished business" that needs to be brought to closure. Privacy allows for demonstrations of physical affection and intimacy.
Determine whether or not the patient embraces a religious faith. If the patient chooses, arrange for clergy visits and encourage expression of spiritual beliefs.	Spiritual beliefs can provide a sense of well-being and hope.
Utilize humor appropriately. Provide cartoons from magazines,	Humor has benefits even for the dying person if used appropriately

Nursing Interventions	Rationales
videotapes, and newspaper clippings that the patient enjoys and can share with the family.	and at the right time. The patient needs to have fun, and laughing with family and friends can be relaxing and can kindle a positive outlook.
Assist the patient and family to "let go" when death is inevitable.	Hope is a vital aspect of living with terminal illness. However, there comes a time when life is over. The patient may be struggling to maintain life for the benefit of the loved ones because they may not know how to let go. The patient and the loved ones may be looking for "permission" to say good-bye.
Provide for the comfort of the loved ones. Encourage their presence and expressions of affection. Remind them that the patient may hear everything that is said even though there is no obvious response.	Families need to know that it is beneficial to communicate intermittently with the patient in soft, gentle tones and to show physical affection through a hug, holding a hand, and kissing.
Continue the physical care of the patient. Allow the family to participate in the care if they so desire.	It is important to the family as well as the patient to know that their loved one is being cared for.

DISCHARGE PLANNING/CONTINUITY OF CARE

If the terminally ill patient is being discharged from hospital to home:
- Arrange for hospice services if patient/family agrees.
- Arrange for other services that may not be provided by hospice: homemaker services, meals-on-wheels, and home health care services.

If the patient is in a long-term care facility:
- Arrange for spiritual services if patient/family agrees.
- Assist family with completing Advance Directives if appropriate.
- Determine whether patient is "do not resuscitate" status. Inform all staff and clarify documentation on medical record.
- Arrange for Social Services to assist patient with financial affairs if necessary.

Table 31.1 • Legal Considerations for Decision Making

Living Will	This document, drawn and signed while the patient is competent, expresses the patient's decisions concerning the administration of life-prolonging medical procedures when there is no chance of regaining a meaningful life. In order for the living will to work, the patient must be in a terminal condition. This document should be reinforced with the Durable Power of Attorney for Health Care document (Illinois Department of Public Health, 1991).
Do-not-resuscitate orders (DNR)	Physician's orders which tell nursing and facility staff that certain measures designed to keep the patient alive are not to be done if the patient suffers cardiopulmonary arrest. In most states, cardiopulmonary resuscitation (CPR) must be started unless there is an order to the contrary in the patient's chart. The DNR orders are consistent with other Advance Directives but are not substitutes for them.
Durable Power of Attorney for Health Care	The patient (principal) can delegate to a person of his or her choice (agent) the power to become his or her agent for any health care decision he or she is unable to make. The agent, not necessarily an attorney, will speak for the patient and make decisions according to the patient's wishes even during periods of physical or mental incapacity. The patient can specify the time which the Durable Power of Attorney will begin and terminate. Unless stated otherwise, the document continues until death (Illinois Department of Public Health, 1991).
Durable Power of Attorney for Property	The patient (principal) can delegate to a person of his or her choice (agent) the power to become his or her agent for financial decisions when the patient becomes incapacitated.
Health care surrogate	If the patient lacks decisional capacity, has a "qualifying condition," and does not have an operative Living Will or Durable Power of Attorney for Health Care, a surrogate is selected from a statutory hierarchy to make decisions regarding life-sustaining treatment.
	NOTE: This varies among states and not all states have Health Care Surrogate legislation (Illinois Department of Public Health, 1991).

Table 31.1 • *continued*

Guardianship	Guardianship is initiated when an individual (other than the patient) petitions the civil court. The allegedly incompetent person, the petitioner, and anyone who would be entitled to be an heir of the estate attend a competency hearing. After hearing evidence, the judge decides incompetency based on the criteria of that state. If the individual is declared incompetent, the judge assigns a guardian to oversee the person and/or that person's estate. The guardian may be a family member, attorney, government agency, or a professional specializing in this work. If plenary guardianship is assigned, the guardian has total legal authority over estate and person. The incapacitated person no longer has the rights of an adult (Stevenson and Capezuti, 1991).

BIBLIOGRAPHY

Editors. (1991). Meeting the challenge of a dying patient. *Nursing 91, 21*(2), 42–46.

Illinois Department of Public Health (1991). *Advance Directives and the Health Care Surrogate Act.* Springfield, IL: Illinois Department of Public Health.

Lillis, P. P., & Prophit, P. (1991). Keeping hope alive. *Nursing 93, 21*(12), 65–66.

Staff. (1990). Cancer Update 90. *Nursing 90, 20*(4), 61–64.

Stevenson, C., & Capezuti, E. (1991). Guardianship: Protection vs. peril. *Geriatric Nursing, 12*(1), 10–13.

Taylor, P. B., & Ferszt, G. G. (1994). Letting go of a loved one. *Nursing 94, 24*(1), 55–56.

Appendices

$\mathcal{A}$PPENDIX A: SUMMARY OF EXPECTED PHYSIOLOGICAL AND PSYCHOSOCIAL CHANGES RELATED TO AGING

PHYSIOLOGICAL CHANGES

Aging changes occur slowly over a period of years, and individuals tend to adjust and compensate for the alterations. The bold print indicates nursing implications that result from aging changes. These include high-risk complications and changes in function which are not always normal aspects of aging but which can occur readily in the presence of disease.

Integumentary System
- Subcutaneous tissue and elastin fibers diminish, causing the skin to become thinner and less elastic.
- Eccrine, apocrine, and sebaceous glands decrease, resulting in diminished secretions and moisturization, causing pruritus.
  - **High risk for impaired skin integrity**
- Body temperature regulation is impaired due to decreased perspiration.
  - **High risk for altered body temperature**
  - **High risk of hyperthermia**
  - **High risk for hypothermia**
  - **Ineffective thermoregulation**
- Capillary blood flow decreases.
  - **Slower wound healing**
  - **High risk for infection**
- Blood supply decreases, especially to lower extremities.
  - **High risk for altered tissue perfusion**

- Vascular fragility occurs.
  - –Senile purpura common
- Cutaneous sensitivity to pressure and temperature are altered.
  - –High risk for pressure ulcers and thermal injuries
- Melanin production is reduced, causing gray-white hair.
- Scalp hair thins. Pubic and axillary hair decreases in females but facial hair increases on upper lip and chin.
- Nail growth slows. Nails become more brittle and longitudinal nail ridges form.
  - –Possible diminished self-esteem related to changes in physical appearance

Musculoskeletal System
- Muscle mass and elasticity diminishes, resulting in decreased strength and endurance, prolonging reaction time and disturbing coordination.
- Bone demineralizes, causing skeletal instability and shrinkage of intervertebral disks. The spine is less flexible and spinal curvature may be present.
- Joints undergo degenerative changes, which may cause pain, stiffness, and loss of range-of-motion (ROM).
  - –Impaired physical mobility
  - –High risk for injury
  - –High risk for trauma
  - –Constipation related to lack of exercise
  - –Functional incontinence related to inability to reach bathroom in time
  - –High risk for disuse syndrome related to lack of exercise

Cardiovascular System
- Cardiac output and recovery time decline.
  - –Heart requires more time to return to normal rate after increasing in response to activity
- The heart rate slows with age.
- Blood flow to all organs decreases. The brain and coronary arteries receive a larger volume than other organs.
- Arterial elasticity decreases, causing increased peripheral resistance.
  - –Results in rise in systolic blood pressure and slight increase in diastolic pressure
- Veins dilate and superficial vessels are more prominent.

Respiratory System
- The muscles of respiration become more rigid, causing decreased vital capacity and increased residual capacity of lungs.
- Alveoli thicken, causing less effective gas exchange.
  - –Shortness of breath may occur during times of physical stress
- The cough mechanism is less effective.
  - –High risk for respiratory tract infection

Gastrointestinal System

- Tooth enamel thins.
- Periodontal disease increases and will result in loss of teeth if not treated.
- Taste buds decrease, resulting in loss of appetite.
- Saliva production is less, causing difficulty with mastication and swallowing.
- Gastric emptying is delayed. Food remains in the stomach longer, decreasing the capacity of the stomach and causing a full feeling too soon.
  - **–Altered nutrition: less than body requirements**
  - **–Impaired swallowing**
- The gag reflex is less effective.
  - **–High risk for aspiration**
- Esophageal peristalsis slows and the esophageal sphincter is less efficient, causing delayed entry of food into the stomach.
- Hiatal hernia is more common.
  - **–Indigestion**
- Peristalsis and nerve sensation of the large intestine is decreased.
  - **–Contributes to constipation**
- Diverticulosis increases with age.
  - **–Risk for developing diverticulitis**
- Liver size decreases after age 70.
- Liver enzymes decrease.
  - **–Drug metabolism and detoxification process affected**
- Gall bladder emptying becomes less efficient. Bile is thicker; cholesterol content is increased.
  - **–Increased incidence of gallstones**

Urinary System

- Nephrons decrease, resulting in decreased filtration and gradual decrease in excretory and reabsorptive functions of renal tubules.
- Glomerular filtration rate decreases.
  - **–Decreased renal clearance of drugs**
- Blood urea nitrogen (BUN) increases by 20% by age 70.
  - **–BUN not always accurate indication of kidney function**
  - **–Creatinine clearance test a better index of renal function in elderly**
- Sodium-conserving ability is diminished.
  - **–Increased risk of hyponatremia**
- Bladder capacity decreases.
  - **–Increased frequency of urination and nocturia**
- Renal function increases when lying down.
  - **–May cause a need to void shortly after going to bed**
- Bladder and perineal muscles weaken, causing an inability to empty the bladder, resulting in postvoid residual.
  - **–High risk for urinary tract infection**
  - **–Increased incidence of stress incontinence in females**
- The prostate may hypertrophy.
  - **–Frequency or dribbling of urine**

Neurologic System
- Neurons in the brain decrease, resulting in decreased production of neurotransmitters causing reduction in synaptic transmission.
- Cerebral blood flow and oxygen utilization are decreased.
  - **It takes more time to carry out motor and sensory tasks requiring speed, coordination, balance, and fine motor hand movements. In the absence of pathology, intellect and capacity for learning remain unchanged.**
- Short-term memory may be somewhat diminished without changes in long-term memory.
  - **Risk for altered thought processes during periods of stress caused by infections, other diseases, and relocation**
- Night sleep decreases due to more frequent and longer wakeful periods.
  - **Sleep pattern disturbance**
- Deep tendon reflexes are decreased.

Sensory Alterations

Vision alterations
- The lens is less pliable, causing presbyopia and decreased accommodation. The lens yellows, causing distorted color perception with greens and blues washing out; warm colors are more distinct. Alterations in the lens causes increased incidence of cataracts.
- Pupil size decreases, allowing less light to enter the eye.
- Vitreous humor changes in consistency, causing blurring of vision.
- The retina changes, resulting in delayed ability to adapt to changes in lighting and decreased ability to tolerate glare.
- Changes in the anterior chamber may cause increased pressure of aqueous humor, resulting in glaucoma.
  - **High risk for trauma**
  - **High risk for injury**

Hearing alterations
- The pinna is less flexible. The hairs in the inner ear stiffen and atrophy and cerumen increases.
- Neurons decrease and the blood supply is less. The tissue in the cochlea deteriorates and the ossicles degenerate.
- Presbycusis results from these changes with loss of tone discrimination. Loss of high-frequency tones occurs first.
  - **High risk for injury**
  - **High risk for trauma**
  - **Social isolation**
  - **Self-esteem disturbance**

Smell and taste alterations
- Taste buds decrease and atrophy with diminished sensitivity for taste.
  - **Altered nutrition: less than body requirements**
- Changes in nose receptors cause decreased sensitivity to smell. (Experts do not agree on this.)

–Altered nutrition: less than body requirements
–High risk for injury
–High risk for trauma

Touch alterations

* There is less ability to discriminate temperature and pressure.
  –High risk for injury
  –High risk for trauma

Kinesthesia alterations

* Diminished proprioception causes problems with balance and coordination.
  –High risk for injury
  –High risk for trauma

Immune System

* Autoantibodies increase, resulting in increased incidence of autoimmune disorders.
  –High risk for infection

Endocrine System

* Release of insulin is delayed by the beta cells of the pancreas.
  –Increase in blood glucose
* Changes in the thyroid may lower basal metabolic rate.

Reproductive System: Females

* Estrogen production decreases with onset of menopause.
* Ovaries, uterus, and cervix decrease in size.
* The vagina shortens, narrows, and becomes less elastic with a thinner lining. Secretions decrease and become more alkaline, resulting in increased incidence of atrophic vaginitis. These changes may result in discomfort during coitus.
* Breast tissue decreases and nipple erection is diminished during sexual arousal.
  –Altered sexuality patterns
* Supporting musculature weakens, increasing risk of uterine prolapse.
* Libido remains unchanged.

Reproductive System: Male

* Testosterone production decreases, resulting in decreased size of testicles.
* Sperm count and viscosity of seminal fluid decreases.
* The penis remains softer during erection. More time is required to achieve erection, delaying achievement of orgasm. There is greater control but less intensity of ejaculation.
* Prostate gland may enlarge.
  –Altered sexuality patterns
* Libido remains unchanged.

PSYCHOSOCIAL CHANGES

- Experience of loss of loved ones through death, relocation, divorce, or estrangement
- Disrupted relationships due to losses
- Loss of roles due to losses
- Difficulty socializing because of sensory deficits
- Need to adapt to changing situations related to changes in health status, relationships, and finances
  - **–Social isolation**
  - **–Altered role performance**
  - **–Altered family processes**
  - **–Caregiver role strain**
  - **–Altered sexuality patterns**
  - **–Grieving**

When planning care, always assess and utilize the patient's strengths. Examples:

- free of deficits or impairments or has successfully adapted to or is adequately compensating for the deficit or impairment
- cognitively healthy
- healthy life-style
- adequate functional ability to carry out activities of daily living (ADL) and to be independent
- free of incapacitating physical discomfort
- lives in physically safe environment
- knowledgeable and realistic about capabilities
- compliant with health care regime
- intact support system, cohesive family unit
- satisfying relationships with others
- opportunities for sexual expression
- access to transportation
- relinquishes roles as phases of life require and replaces them with satisfying new roles
- pattern of successful mourning for losses
- participates in groups
- utilizes successful problem-solving skills
- self-confident in abilities and judgment
- makes decisions and accepts responsibilities for decisions
- well-defined value system
- accepts what cannot be changed
- finds comfort and strength in spiritual beliefs
- participates in healthy reminiscing and has few regrets for past life
- finds meaning and enjoyment in hobbies and activities
- experiences joy in nature, art, and music and has well-developed sense of humor

APPENDIX B: HOME ENVIRONMENTAL SAFETY ASSESSMENT

Eliminate
- Throw rugs
- Furniture from walkways
- Electrical cords and wires from walkway
- Waxed floors
- Glare from lights, waxed floors

Suggest
- Adequate nonglare lighting
- Night lights in bathroom and bedroom
- Painting edges of curbs and steps in contrasting color
- Placing treads on steps
- Installing grab bars in tub/shower
- Placing chair in tub/shower
- Slip-proof mats in tub/shower
- Installing hand-held shower
- Installing raised toilet seat
- Solid chairs with sturdy arm rests
- Handrails for stairs

Check
- Electrical outlets
- Electrical equipment grounded
- Fuse boxes
- Temperature of hot water heater and radiators
- Use of smoking materials
- Refrigerator for spoiled food
- Ability to use stove safely
- Chemicals for correct labels
- Medications for correct labels

- Use of candles, matches
- Patient's ability to hear telephone, doorbell
- Patient's ability to smell spoiled food, gas, fire

NOTE: See Chapter 21, page 207 for additional safety considerations for cognitively impaired individuals.

APPENDIX C: TEACHING ELDERLY PATIENTS

- Individuals learn only if they perceive a need for learning and are willing to invest the time and energy required. For the elderly, disabled patient, energy resources are limited so appropriate timing is essential.
- Consider the patient's values, interests, activities, and life-style. Explain to the patient how to meet health care needs within the current life-style. For example, tell the diabetic how he or she can still travel and eat in restaurants.
- The patient may not perceive present health status as a problem. The patient may have multiple problems and may prioritize them differently than the caregivers.
- Find out what the patient already knows. Evaluate the accuracy of present knowledge. Misconceptions may have to be cleared up before other teaching begins.
- Take advantage of every teaching opportunity. Answer questions as they arise.
- Start with simple information and build to more complex instruction. Teach only what the patient needs to know. If a stroke patient has a permanent housekeeper, he or she does not need to learn how to adapt cooking skills using the strong arm.
- The person in a nursing home who views the placement as preparation for death may see no need for learning. Patients in nursing homes or in their own homes may feel that the staff or family members will assume the responsibility of their welfare and see no need for learning. Include the family if possible so they can reinforce the instructions.
- Occasionally a patient and family feel that staff is getting paid to provide services that the patient is capable of performing independently. The nurse is a key factor in altering these beliefs. The nurse must believe in the program and have the knowledge and skills to effectively deliver the instruction and evaluate patient progress.

- Attend to the patient's physical and safety needs before initiating the teaching/learning process. Physical discomfort related to hunger, elimination needs, or pain makes learning impossible. Arrange an environment with a comfortable temperature, free from stress, distractions, and noise.
- The patient's trust and respect for the nurse enhance the learning progress. Build on the patient's upper level needs. The person who is learning feels increased esteem, and in turn this increases the desire to learn and succeed. Offer feedback, encouragement, and praise when appropriate.
- Consider sensory deficits. Remind the patient to insert the hearing aid or put on glasses if necessary. Adapt teaching methods and materials to the patient's deficits. Use a variety of methods if possible: seeing, hearing, touching, and doing.
- Evaluate the patient's mental status, especially attention span, short-term memory, response time, and ability to concentrate. Do not attempt to accomplish too much at one time. Individuals learn at their own speed and older adults may take longer to learn and carry out a particular task. Know the patient's abilities and limitations and monitor for signs of physical and mental fatigue.
- Evaluate the communication skills of the patient. If there is a language impairment, consult with the speech pathologist to adapt the teaching accordingly.
- Write all specific directions on the care plan so teaching methods are consistent. Document the patient's progress.
- The patient's progress is not always continuous or consistent. There are numerous variables which can influence the patient's performance on any given day. Do not give up the intervention or the patient because of a failure. If, over a period of time, it is evident that the intervention is ineffective, then reassessment is indicated.
- Teach skills for activities of daily living at the time the task is normally carried out; for example, teach feeding skills at meal time. Remember that many different steps are required to complete a specific activity of daily living. Review the functional assessment to determine the reason for the self-care deficit and which steps the patient cannot complete. The patient may not have the potential for completing every step, but give the patient the opportunity to reach an optimal level, with assistance provided as necessary.
- If adaptive aids or assistive devices are necessary for completion of an activity, give instructions to the patient in the use of such equipment. Avoid problems by including the instructions on the care plan. The patient must find the equipment aesthetically acceptable and be willing to use it.
- Learning is hard work at best and requires the cooperation and efforts of the staff, the patient, and the family. Avoid placing too much emphasis on success. Accept the patient at the current level and administer frequent doses of tender loving care with the instruction.

BIBLIOGRAPHY

Cordell, B., & Smith-Blair, N. (1994). Streamlined charting for patient education. *Nursing 94, 24*(1), 57–59.

Cunningham, D. (1993). Improving your teaching skills. *Nursing 93, 23*(12), 24j.

Dellasega, C., et al. (1994). Teaching elderly clients. *Journal of Gerontological Nursing, 20*(1), 31–38.

Stewart, K. B., & Walton, R. L. (1992). Teaching the elderly. *Nursing 92, 22*(10), 66, 68.

Weinrich, S. P., Boyd, M., & Nussbaum, J. (1989). Continuing education: Adapting strategies to teach the elderly. *Journal of Gerontological Nursing, 15*(11), 17–21.

APPENDIX D: MINI MENTAL STATUS EXAMINATION (MMSE)

1. *Orientation to time*
   Ask for date. Then ask for specific parts omitted. One point for each correct answer.
   Year _____ Season _____ Date _____ Day _____ Month _____
   (5) _____
   Orientation to place
   Ask "Where are we now?" Then ask for specifics. One point for each correct answer.
   State ___ County _____ City ___ Hospital _____ Floor _____
   (5) _____

2. *Registration*
   Tell the patient you have three words you want him or her to remember. Say the words apple, elephant, and chair. Ask the patient to repeat the words. Score one point for each word. If not correct, repeat the words, and then ask the patient to do the same up to six trials. If more than one trial is needed, record number here _____.
   (3) _____

3. *Attention*
   Serial 7's. Ask patient to begin with 100 and count backward by 7. Stop after five subtractions (93, 86, 79, 72, 65). Score equals number correct. If patient refuses, ask him or her to spell *world* backward. Score equals number of letters in correct order, e.g., dlrow=5, dlorw=3.
   (5) _____

4. *Recall*
   Ask for three objects repeated above. One point each.
   (3) _____

5. *Language*
   Naming Ask resident to name *watch*, then *pencil*. One point each.
   (2) _____

Repetition Repeat this: No if's, and's, or but's.
(1) _____
Command Hold up a piece of paper and say "Take this piece of paper in your right hand, fold it in half, and put it on the floor." Three points; circle the correct stages.
(3) _____
Read Show patient a card with "close your eyes" printed on it. Ask him or her to read it and do what it says. One point.
(1) _____
Write Ask patient to write a complete sentence on a piece of paper. Must contain subject and verb and be sensible; correct grammar and punctuation not necessary. One point.
(1) _____
Copying Ask resident to copy design. All 10 angles must be present and the designs must intersect. Tremor, rotation ignored. One point.
(1) _____
(30) Total Score_____

Adopted from J. Psych. Research 12: 189–198 (1975) with kind permission from Elsevier Science Ltd., The Boulevard, Langford Lane, Kidlington OX5 1GB, UK.

INDEX

Tables are indicated by *t*.

A

Above-the-knee amputation (AKA). *See* Lower extremity amputation
Acetaminophen with codeine, 322
Acetic acid, 12
Acetylcholine, 203
Acquired immunodeficiency syndrome (AIDS), 6
  dementia, 217*t*
Actinic keratosis, 35
Active assistive range of motion (AAROM), 248
Active range of motion (AROM), 248
Acute illness, symptoms of, 126
Acyclovir ointment, 8*t*
Adaptive devices for eating, 264
Adult Protective Services, 295
Advance Directives, 325, 329, 330
Aerobic exercise, 90
Afterload, 75
Age-related macular degeneration, 283
Agnosia, 204, 212, 225
Agranulocytosis, 140*t*
AIDS. *See* Acquired immunodeficiency syndrome (AIDS)
Alcohol
  and depression, 301
  and elder abuse, 293
Alerting devices for the hearing impaired, 280
Alpha-1-antitrypsin determination, 113
Alpha-1-protease inhibitor, 113
Alzheimer's disease (AD) and related dementias, 129, 136
  acetylcholine, 203
  amyloid beta-protein, 203
  clinical/diagnostic findings, 204
  clinical manifestations, 203–204
  diagnostic criteria for dementia, 218*t*
  discharge planning/continuity of care, 216
  discussion, 203

  etiologies, 203
  major forms of dementia, 217*t*
  Medic-Alert device, 207
  Mini Mental Status Examination (MMSE), 349–350
  nursing diagnosis
    altered family processes, 214–216
    altered thought processes, 204–206
    anxiety, 209–211
    functional incontinence, 209
    high risk for altered nutrition-less than body requirements, 212–213
    high risk for trauma, 206–207
    impaired verbal communication, 211–212
    self-care deficits (grooming and hygiene), 213–214
    sleep pattern disturbance, 208–209
  tacrine, 216
  phenytoin, 214
  safe environment, maintaining, 207
  and sexual dysfunction, 315–316
  sundowning, 208–209
Ambulation, after CVA, 222–223
Amputation
  and PVD, 100
  See also Lower extremity amputation
Amyloid beta-protein, 203
Anaphylactoid reactions, 140*t*
Aneurysm, 97
Ankle-foot orthosis (AFO), 249
Ankylosis, 71*t*, 248
Anorexia, 141*t*
Anthropometric measurements, 16
Anticholinergic medicine, 170
Anticipatory grieving, 242–243
Anticoagulants, 109
Anticonvulsants, 140*t*
Antidepressants, 5
Antiplatelet agents, 109
Antipruritic emollient, 29